Only a mother could love him

ADD: Attention Deficit Disorder

Ben Polis

Inquiries should be made to:
Seaview Press
PO Box 234
Henley Beach, South Australia 5022
Telephone: 61 8 8235 1535
Fax: 61 8 8235 9144
Email: seaview@seaviewpress.com.au

Cover by Brett Warren at www.capturedesign.com.au

Cartoons by Jessica Simeon

www.addhelpguide.com site designed by Glenn Cook,
TTR Web Design www.ttrwebdesign.com

National Library of Australia Cataloguing-in-Publications entry
Polis, Benjamin, 1981-
Only a mother could love him : ADD : attention deficit disorder

ISBN 1 74008 169 2

1. Polis, Benjamin, 1981- 2. Attention-deficit-disorder
children – Biography 3. Attention-deficit hyperactivity disorder
Popular works.
1. Title

616.85890092

Dedication

This book is dedicated to my parents, for without
them I would have achieved little …

Special thanks ..

I would like to offer my sincerest thanks to Glenn Cook from **TTR Web Design** for enabling my website design to be so user friendly, keeping it up to date, and always available for my computer support. **TTR Web Design** offers more than just a web site design and hosting, they offer exceptional customer service that would be hard to beat. At any given time, be it day or night, I am able to call for assistance in either updating my current website or asking questions in relation to my computer software or hardware. Their vast knowledge of computer systems is extraordinary. Only recently I was able to work until 3.30 am with Glenn on updating my e-book and changes to my existing book cover. You certainly not get service like that from your average design house. Rarely do I not get an immediate answer to any query I may have and I thoroughly recommend **TTR Web Design** to anyone who may be thinking of updating or having a site designed and hosted by **TTR Web Design.**

Of course, I could go to the various people that have helped me in the past with my book, but I *know,* that when I contact **TTR Web Design,** the job will be done professionally and efficiently to my sometimes ridiculous time constraints.

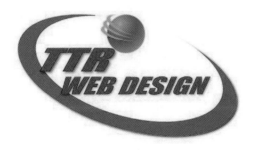

www.ttrwebdesign.com

Acknowledgments

I would like to thank the following people who helped me with this book:

Henry and Gaye Polis (my parents) who put up with me over the years and especially while writing this book. Dr. Luk (my childhood psychiatrist) who helped me understand my ADD. Aunty Anne and Uncle Phillip, thank you for your help with the proof reading, etc. My Year 10 teacher for adding his opinion and words of wisdom to this book. Glenn Cook and Tony Harrington for developing my web site and answering my sometimes stupid computer questions. Brett Warren for designing the front cover and Jessica Simeon for the fantastic cartons.

I would also like to thank the following people who had an impact on my life:

Gaye Polis, for being the best mum in the world. I have made it this far, Mum, and I owe a lot to you for my success. You were always there for me when I needed you most. I love you, Mum!

Henry Polis, for being a great dad. We may not see eye to eye on a lot of things but I respect you and love you dearly. If I grow up to be half the man you are I will be a great man. I love you, too, Dad!

Adelaide Polis: We have never been good friends for obvious reasons, but you will always be my favorite and only sister. In the future I hope we can settle our differences and become close friends as brother and sister.

Tess Polis (my dog): You have spent many hours with me while writing this book. You never complained when the stereo was up loud or it was too late at night and you wanted to go to sleep. You never complained when I was in a bad mood and were always ready for a hug. As my mother would say, "Teeeeesssssssss!"

Aunty Anne Scott: I have always seen you as a second mother to me. You have helped me on so many occasions I could never list them all. Thank you for helping me get into university!

Uncle Phillip Scott: For taking me to my first Australian Rules Football match and for our countless hours of conversation on sports. I admire and look up to you as both a friend and an uncle.

Aunty Susanne Boak: Thank you for your support. I will always remember my first hicky, which you gave me on my 13th birthday.

Uncle Campbell Boak: I may not have agreed with your choice in football teams but I agree with a lot of other people's opinion of you. You were a great man, the gentle giant and I miss you. I think about you all the time! If I ever needed a talk you were always there to listen. So many times you caught me doing naughty things on the trains but you never told anyone. You always stuck up for me when other people didn't. Thank you for the great memories. I love you Uncle Campbell!

My Year 10 teacher: You always pointed me in the right direction, sometimes pushing me against my will. In the letter you gave me on the last day of school in Year Ten you told me to "never sell yourself short." I hope I have not sold myself short and disappointed a man I respect so much.

My Year Nine teacher: You stuck up for me when other people wanted to expel me from school (again). You went in to bat for me over and over and I never really understood until I wrote this book that without you I might not have come this far. Thank you!

My Grade Two teacher: I have very fond memories of you even though many years have passed. You were the one who recognized that I had reading problems and helped me learn to read. Without you I may still be spelling "of" as "ov."

My principal in Year Ten: You always knew what the boys were up to, especially me. I respect you for what you have done for me, but more importantly, for all the boys' lives you touch every day by being their teacher and friend.

My principal in Grades One to Grade Three: You recognized that I was a little bit different and not like everyone else, but you never held that against me.

Mrs. N: You taught me that you can only push so hard before something breaks. You are a great person and a great teacher. We nearly made it!

Mr. K: Thank you for teaching me that there are some teachers out there who have mastered the art of capturing the elusive concentration of an ADD student. I always left your class with a smile and a sense of time well spent. Your sometimes different learning styles really captured and fueled my thirst and love for economics. I learned much more than economic principles from you. You taught me that if you make any topic fun and exciting you can really reach students. You are one of the best teachers I have ever experienced. More important than that, you are a caring and kind man and you do not receive the praise you deserve.

Mrs. A: What can I say? You are a lovely woman and great teacher. Who would have thought that religious studies would be one of my best subjects? I hope you enjoyed our theological arguments.

Mrs. S: You always surprised me by how happy you were at eight o'clock in the morning. You always try to find good in people.

Tate Patching: You have always stuck by me, mate, when other people haven't. You are one of my closest friends and always will be. I feel the reason we are such good friends is because we have a mutual respect for each other. I could always count on you for a hand with anything. I will always remember my first car with fond memories. You are the cheapest car stereo installer in the world. I remember paying you for three days' work with a $7 sandwich! Another fond memory is when you told me that you could smell petrol in the trunk after I installed the amplifier and I said you were imagining it. Then at the top of your lungs you yelled, "You drilled a hole through the petrol tank, you dick, I quit!" Thanks, Tate, you're a great person and a great friend.

Andrew Stevens: You have been my longest friend and sometimes only friend. We have had some crazy times together, especially in our teenage years.

Grady Patching: My fondest memories of you are of packing my pants when you drove us to parties. You also saved me from having the living daylights beaten out of me. You are a big man but your heart is even bigger.

Dr. Luk: You have been my psychiatrist since I was twelve. You have helped me understand myself more than anyone and helped me through the bad times to the present good times. You are a man to be admired. You love your work but don't do it for any recognition. I have never met anyone like you before and never met a doctor who cares as much as you do. You are a very special person.

Thom Hartmann: You opened my eyes to a different perception of ADD.

Spencer McArtney: You may only be eight years old but I see myself in you every day. We have had some great times together. You brighten up my day even when you barge into my room when I am sleeping. You don't even realize it but you helped with this book. You are a great kid and a great friend.

Contents

Introduction

When I was seventeen I was first asked to write this book on my personal experiences of suffering from Attention Deficit Disorder (ADD). I did not give the idea a second thought. The answer was a plain and simple—"No!" I did not want to talk about it. I didn't even want to think about my personal experiences with ADD.

Why I did not want to write this book was that I was sick and tired of always being looked upon as that "crazy little child" who seemed to be a burden on everyone. My school life was hell, not just for me, but for my parents as well. Not to mention the teachers who I challenged every day in the classroom. I hated the fact that I was different and at times even hated myself for who I was and what I was doing.

When gathering my research material from the many schools where I was a student, I was embarrassed by a lot of the terrible things I had done. But at the time I did not know what I was doing. I was often confused, not understanding what I was doing. This caused a lot of depression in my early school days. As I got older it became a lot easier to deal with my problem. I overcame it in a number of ways including medication and self-taught techniques that I will discuss in greater detail in later chapters.

Looking back on my short life at the age of nineteen now, it all

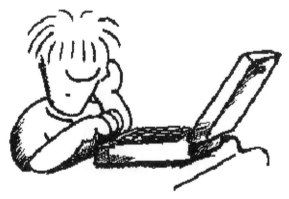

seems like a far away story when I recall these things in my life. I still have no idea why I did these things that normal society sees as abnormal. If you or your child has ADD you will understand what I mean when I say abnormal behavior—those fits of anger and impulsive behavior that are unleashed on family members and which seem to have no reason or specific purpose. It must be very hard for parents to deal with and understand why their child is behaving in this abnormal manner. This book, I hope, will help you understand why your child acts in this uncontrolled way.

It was not until I turned nineteen that I seriously considered the challenge of writing this book. After watching a story on children with ADD on the Channel 9 program *Sixty Minutes*, I felt that I had to write this book to help other people suffering what I have endured throughout my life. However, again I put it off! One day it will happen, I thought to myself. I didn't have the time, I had study at university and I was going out all the time. But it was really just an excuse. I just didn't care enough, I guess.

A young boy down the road has ADD. For the past couple of years my mother has been saying, "Why don't you go talk to the boy's mother?" I usually brushed it aside with, "Yeah, maybe later." Then one day I decided to talk to the mother and she was pretty upset with her son's progress at school because he was behind in reading and math, etc. This was a shock to me. I did not understand what she was worried about because I could not read a short sentence until I was in Grade Five. I told her this, along with other personal experiences. It always seems to surprise people when I tell them things about my life at school and home. They often look at me with amazement and even confusion. I believe this is because now I do not act like a *freak*, as my sister called me. However, I can understand where this confusion comes from. If you'd said to my parents when I was ten, "Your son will pass Year Twelve and pass it well," they would probably have bet their house that this would not happen, or that their child would go on to university and write a book—they would have probably bet their lives on that not happening. Well, it did and this book will tell you about the remarkable turnaround in my life and I hope it will help your child achieve the best results possible.

I have no accredited medical knowledge of ADD. However, I do not understand how so-called medical experts develop theories and strategies for parents with children with ADD. Their advice is often very useful. But how can they really understand it without actually living with someone who has ADD or having it themselves? I am not knocking the medical experts because my doctor is an excellent one and does understand ADD in great depth. The strategies that I developed were invaluable in my remarkable turnaround from very possibly ending up in a child detention center to making it to university.

However, I have skimmed through many books on this topic and at times it makes me very angry because these books are often filled with medical mumbo-jumbo that really does not help with the treatment of your child with ADD. They do help partly in understanding what ADD is, in a medical sense, which is always a good start for parents. But techniques and strategies are often not found in these books. I searched in many libraries and on the

Internet to find a book by a young person who has ADD, and I could not find one. The closest I found was a book written by an American author which included personal experiences written by college students. This was a surprise to me. I could not believe that someone had not written a book on their experiences and how they overcame their problems in everyday situations. Well now someone has and I guess it's about time!

This book will not give the answer to all the problems you will come across in managing your child's condition, but it will help. Many parents feel isolated. They feel depression, confusion, and a sense of blame—and of course anger and frustration. My parents have lost a number of friends throughout my life as a result of my behavior. People would not invite my parents to parties and gatherings because I would cause too many problems. Along with this, my parents would cut themselves off from people because they were embarrassed by my behavior. My dad told me that they were invited to a lot of gatherings, but only once! Narrow-minded people who did not understand would often make comments such as, "Leave him with me and I will give him a good belting and pull him in line." My parents were often accused of being bad parents who could not control their son. This was not true, because I have a sister two years older than me. She is the most polite and nicest person you could ever meet. In my younger years my parents took me to see a number of psychiatrists who said it was my parents' fault and that there was nothing wrong with me. How wrong they were!

Now, getting back to the little boy I am tutoring. After offering my services to the mother with his schoolwork I was quite worried the first time I went to their house. I did not know what to expect. I thought I might have bitten off more than I could chew. Well, the first day I went over there the mother showed me his schoolwork, which was simple word games to promote word recognition.

It often took the mother over an hour to get him to do it. This hour was mostly taken up with erratic behavior including swearing, yelling—basically everything except doing his homework. The first time I went over to their house it took me only fifteen minutes. I had promised to play a game of Nintendo with him afterwards. He had done his work and he knew it and was playing his Nintendo. The mother told him to get up and do his homework. I told her that he had done it and done it twice. This was accomplished without medication through techniques I have developed while suffering from this condition. I get great pleasure out of helping people with this problem. I enjoy it more because I know how isolated these children feel at school and at home. These techniques and strategies will be discussed in greater detail in later chapters.

I will discuss a number of issues in this book, including picking the right school for your child, and the teacher, if possible. This is of great concern to me because I went to six schools and I know what works and what doesn't.

I will talk about other areas: parenting techniques, including anger management; homework, which can be basically impossible for some parents; discipline, what works and what will never work. I know my parents tried everything: medication, which is always a hot topic in the ADD network; relationships between parents and siblings and the child with ADD. These are just a couple of issues that I will discuss. I hope that you will find this book as useful in the management of your child as I believe you will. I would just like to add that this book will be most useful only if you are prepared to put in lots of tiring and frustrating hours of work with your child!

I wish you and your child the greatest success in overcoming this problem.

Benjamin Polis

0 to 4

I, Benjamin Heinrich Polis, was born at Sandringham Hospital, Melbourne, Australia on the 7th of August 1981. On this day the angels sang out aloud, "What have we done?"

My life had just started, but for my parents, it changed theirs forever. I was a healthy looking baby with no obvious physical or mental problems. My parents were pleased that I was "normal." It is what all parents hope for in their newborn child. But they were in for a rude shock! My hidden handicap would not be discovered until many years later. Looking back on my early years, my parents have told me there were a number of things that appeared to be unusual in my behavior. Of course I do not remember much, so this information has been recounted by parents and family members.

My mother told me she was not able to breastfeed me in a room with other people in it. Any movement or object in the room would distract me. I would stop feeding and gaze around the room searching for some other source of entertainment. She overcame this by always removing me to another room. It was the first of many times throughout my life I was to be separated or banned from my own age group. Thinking back, it was probably the first time my parents experienced my short attention span and how easily distracted I was, the classic or common signs of ADD. I still have these symptoms today and probably will for the rest of my life, but now I understand the problem and I can control my behavior.

Some people refer to the terrible twos as the age when babies start to crawl and begin walking. I can imagine the first time I started to walk, loving the freedom and thinking "Let's bust out of this place!" Well, that's just what I did, all the time, every time. For me, any room was no barrier, just another challenge. I always found

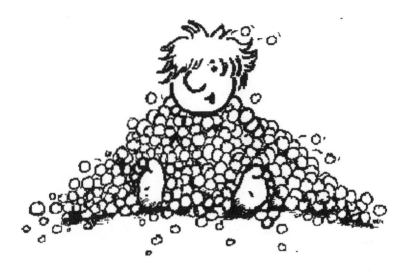

some ingenious way to bust out and explore this new and exciting world. My mother talks about frequently losing me, searching high and low until she found me, until next time when she would start the search again. My father recalls coming home from work to find my mother vacuuming the backyard. I had opened up a beanbag and covered the entire backyard with white polystyrene balls. Hey, I wanted a white Christmas!

Ash Wednesday 1983

Bushfires raged across Victoria and South Australia. This was one of the scariest days in my parents' life. My father remembers looking at the Melbourne horizon and seeing a ring of fire and smoke. It was the first time my parents experienced childhood asthma. They were in a state of panic with their two-year-old child who had begun gasping for breath. Dad rushed me to Frankston Hospital. It was eerie. The streets were deserted as people stayed at home. The air-conditioning in the car was sucking in the smoke while I sucked and gasped for life-giving air. Two or three times a year there were high-speed car trips to hospital, where I had to stay one to three weeks, with nurses watching me all the time. My asthma became worse as I got older. At about ten I was rushed from Frankston Hospital to the Royal Children's Hospital in an ambulance, accompanied by a specialist doctor and nurse. I was in intensive care for days with a collapsed lung. My parents were not told at first of the collapsed lung.

I remember one day very clearly. The specialist doctor pulled his chair close to me and said, "If you don't start to look after yourself and take your daily asthma medication you will be dead in two years." Believe me, from that day I have taken my asthma medication. Looking back, I believe the reason that my parents were not told of the severity of my condition was because the doctors were trying to look after not just me but my parents as well. I remember so many incidents when I would call out to my parents in the middle of the night and tell them that I wanted or needed to go to hospital. I hated going to hospital but always knew it was the best place for me. Without the excellent care of the staff at both Frankston and the Royal Children's Hospital, I would be dead. So I would like to thank them for all they have done for me and all other sick children.

One problem arose time and time again. When I became better I could not sit still, a well-recognized symptom of ADD. The doctors would say, "Ben should be right to go home in a couple of days." I would get excited and work myself up so much that I did more harm than good. I would rip the intravenous drip out of my vein, jump out of bed, run to the cafeteria to buy a Coke and lollies then run through the wards and back to my bed. This made me sick again, often worse than before. Then I would be told that I could not go home yet. Confused and angry, I would cry, throw a whopper of a temper tantrum, throw my pillows and food at the nurses, rip up my medical charts and so on. My parents would be upset by my bad behavior but could do nothing. Their little boy wanted to go home but they could not take him because he most probably would die. What a terrible position for my parents, or any parents, to be in! My father would often smuggle in a McDonald's burger to cheer me up.

The Children's Hospital was thirty-five kilometers from home and with the long hours they were working to establish their own real-estate business, it was hard for my parents to see me, but they did. I was scared, confused and bored sitting in a hospital bed with tubes in my veins and asthma medication pumped into me every ten minutes. I hated being in hospital. Then one day my father told me, "Grow up, this is the best place for you. You are lucky you don't have diabetes and need insulin shots four times a day." I guess this was the first time I looked at myself in a positive new light. I thought to myself, "Hey, you're sick but you're luckier than a lot of other kids." This positive thought process would be transferred to my ADD handicap later in life, especially during my teen years. After I finally accepted that I had ADD, and needed to work around it and use it to my advantage, my life became a lot easier.

We lived on a long and busy road. I would climb anything to escape, then run like the wind up the road with my mother in hot pursuit. If she were watching our front yard too closely, then it would be out the back door, over the fence, into the neighbor's house through their doggie door and out through their front door—free again!

As I got older and stronger my climbing abilities became greater and more daring. I could always climb fences but now I would even climb over the roof to escape. I could climb anything and would jump from any height. This is a characteristic of ADD children.

They act impulsively, not thinking, even for a brief moment, of the consequences of their actions. Remarkably, I have never broken any bones, but it is interesting to note that ADD children are the largest contributors, as a percentage, to broken-bone injuries in juveniles. My advice to parents is to form a good relationship with your doctor. You will need it.

My greatest climbing achievement was when I was about three. My mother loved to sew and would drag me to every fabric store in Melbourne. For hour after hour she would flick through pattern books and study fabrics while I ran amok through the large stores. I hated those stores, I still hate them and refuse to go into them, even today. However, I always found a way to amuse myself. I usually sat and climbed over the large material rolls. My mother laughs as she tells me she loved it when I got lost. She deliberately lost me sometimes so she would get some peace and quiet shopping, then she would find me when she was finished.

But one particular day was very different. I climbed on the outside of the escalator all the way to the top, shuffling my feet along a small shelf on the outside of the escalator. The only problem was, I could not get down. This time I do remember telling myself that I was not going to jump. Five meters below me was a hard concrete floor. My mother (still looking at those bloody patterns) was found and got into a state of panic. From all over the store, people gathered to look at me with fear and amazement, probably thinking, "How did that kid get up there?" They stopped the escalator and someone brought me down. That was the first and last time I climbed an escalator. But harder and higher structures were soon on the drawing board.

Around age four, my behavior became more destructive and erratic. My grandparents took me to the Royal Melbourne Zoo for a picnic. I ran off to explore. Both grandparents were not worried because I was still in sight and safe. Well, let me rephrase that. I was safe but the people having nice quiet picnics were not. It was a lovely fine sunny day. I had found liquid gold at the end of the rainbow, the main tap to the extensive watering system for the lawns. With a couple of twists the sprinklers opened up and the entire picnic area was sprayed with water. I ran off leaving a path of destruction in my wake. It took many minutes before the staff turned off the sprinkler system, but it was too late, everyone's picnic had been flooded. Don't you love Melbourne's unpredictable weather? After that, my grandparents hardly ever took me anywhere. I guess I know why.

On our long road lived an old, scruffy, brownish red dog. Hour after hour this dog would lie across the concrete footpath basking in the hot sun. I hated that dog. Mum and Dad had given me my first bike and I loved it! It gave me freedom and an even faster escape than my little legs. I have fond memories of this bike. I remember every little detail about it. It was bright yellow with a long black seat, in a classic sixties chopper style. I had put on a couple of minor improvements—noisy plastic beads on the wheel spokes, plus a big red flag on a fibreglass pole for safety. But I believe this was for other people's safety not mine—"Here I come, get out of my way!"

Anyway, back to the dog. I would ride all day up and down the footpath in front of our house. On our neighbor's driveway was a ramp made from the curve in the guttering. I would ride like a bat out of hell up the road and then make a quick turn onto the ramp to get some airtime. The only problem was that this dog would sunbake on my landing strip. I constantly had to swerve to miss both him and the tree next to him. I crashed many times but always got straight back on my bike and did it all over again.

The dog was my arch-enemy, but not for long! This day was going to be very different! It was either the dog or me. I made a plan that at the time I thought was foolproof. How wrong I was!

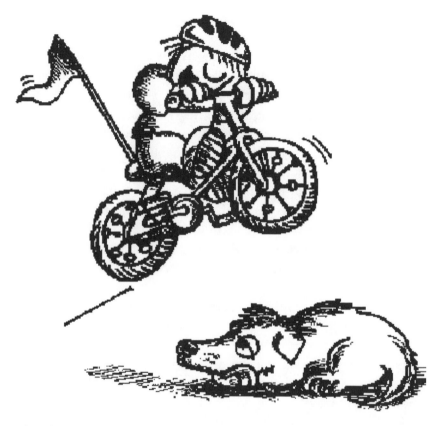

The plan went something like this. I rode all the way to the end of the street, some hundred meters in length. I turned the great yellow chopper around and started to ride as fast as my four-year-old legs would let me. I was instantly transformed into that famous motorcycle stunt rider, the Great Evel Knievel. The plan was that the dog would be so scared it would quickly move when it saw me coming right for it. Up the ramp I went, faster and higher than ever before. The dog lazily opened one eye and saw me coming but just lay there, until the yellow chopper and I landed right on him, crushing his ribs. The dog had to be put down, though I suspect some people would say it would have been more fitting for me to be put down!

Thinking and talking about this now is very painful for me. I have no idea why I did it and I am not proud of it. The only explanation I can give is that my impulsiveness once again got the better of me. I could blame it on my ADD but I never have and never will use my ADD as an excuse for my actions. Today, I understand that this is the way I am and I can now control my actions. When I was younger, it was nearly impossible. My mother recalls buying flowers for the dog's owner. Over the years, my mother and the florist shop lady had a very good relationship. My mother said, "I kept her in business." Time after time she would buy flowers for people and apologize for the things I had done. It was even more embarrassing for her when some people received flowers more than once.

At kindergarten, my parents first experienced the constant embarrassment in having me as their child. Every day my mother would pick me up and every day she would be bombarded with stories from both the teacher and the parents of the other children. "Ben did this!" and "Ben did that!" Mum hated picking me up; the emotional strain was often too much to handle. This is a regular problem for parents of ADD children. They love their child, but it can be so tiring to continually defend them against accusations from other adults. Sometimes the strain of defending their child becomes too much and the parents' love turns into frustration, then to anger. Asking or yelling at the child, "Why did you do that?" will achieve nothing. I did not know my behavior was unacceptable and neither will your child. I also hated kindergarten because I was always in trouble. I was often confused and suffered from low self-esteem, because I did not know what I was doing wrong. In my mind I was acting normally—my idea of normal, not other people's opinion of normal. I would sit by the entrance, often crying uncontrollably while I waited for my mother. I always knew when she was coming to save me because I could smell her distinctive perfume.

The kindergarten soon got sick of me (like many other schools in my life) and I pretty much stopped going. When I asked my mother about going to kindergarten, she laughed and said, "You hardly went there!" I stopped due to an incident with a mentally disabled child. The boy was autistic and would strangle people for no reason. Thinking about that now, I guess he did have a reason, we just didn't know what it was. One day this boy strangled and bit me. So I did what any ADD child would have done. I strangled him back and bit him harder than he had. I got into so much trouble I refused to go back and I am sure they were pleased with that! The problem for parents is that if their child has an easily recognizable condition, for example autism, mental disability, whatever, then the child's actions are understood and excused. But if the child is suffering from ADD then it is labeled as bad or uncontrollable and the parents are to blame. All I can say to parents is, keep loving your child. Things will get better as the child grows older and learns to control their behavior and actions.

Around this time I started seeing child and family psychiatrists. Mum and Dad called them the family doctors to nicen it up a bit. I now realize they were embarrassed and trying to hide the fact that their child needed psychiatric help. The whole family would go along: Gaye, my mother, Henry, my father, Adelaide, my sister, and me. We would all sit around a big room and talk about our problems. I hated talking about our problems because it was always something to do with me. I felt as though they should have just said, "Hey, Ben, you're the problem," and tattooed it on my head. The doctors would talk to every family member individually, then talk about our problems again, trying to find a solution. We went every Friday to our "family doctor," month after month, year after year.

"What is wrong with him?" my parents would ask. The most common answer was: "Nothing, it's just bad parenting techniques, basically you're just bad parents. You'd better come back next Friday so we can talk about this in more detail."

Looking back, I guess it was not the doctors' fault and definitely not my parents'. Our problem was ADD, which was not as widely recognized or diagnosed as it is today. They couldn't help me because they didn't understand the problem. Unlike today, there were no help groups or books to help parents understand. It was not until I was twelve that I was diagnosed with ADHD (Attention Deficit Hyperactivity Disorder) and received some useful medical help. My parents often felt helpless, not knowing why their child was so upset about everything and everyone. My mother recalls crying herself to sleep on many nights wondering, "What can I do? Maybe we are bad parents as the doctors told us." We struggled on as a family, fighting, yelling at each other and basically just not working as a "normal" family unit.

The best time of my life. Prep! Yeah, right!

For most children, school is a time of great excitement and happiness, but not for me, my parents, or the teachers in the six schools I attended during the next twelve years. I was constantly segregated from the class and sent outside. Reading and writing were definitely not my forte. I struggled with every aspect of school life except finding my way to the principal's office. My first school was the nearby government school and my reputation had come with me, as it still does today. My mother described how on my first day one of the teachers greeted us with, "So you're Ben Polis. We've heard all about you. I hope you're not going to cause trouble here." What had they heard about me? Who told them? Was it the kindergarten teachers, was it the parents of the kindergarten children? I don't know and I would like to say that I don't care. But I do care because from day one I never had a chance at that school. My mother was furious and hurt.

Unfortunately for me, my behavior attracted the wrong attention. I was dared by the other kids to show my boy's bits to a girl. So I went right up to this girl and showed her my bits. They thought I was fantastic. So did I. The girl told the teacher and I was in trouble again. The teacher used reverse psychology on me and asked, "Ben, would you like to show the whole class?" "Okay," I said, and I did. Well, I got into trouble again. ADD children do not understand situations like these until they are older. What their brains tell them to do isn't always the right thing. It takes a lot of embarrassing experiences and a strong will to overcome this major problem of impulsiveness.

Another incident occurred when the school was assembled in the library to sing, dance and participate in Australian folk songs. There were maybe fifty to eighty excited children sitting on the floor talking loudly. A teacher walked in and yelled, "Ben Polis! You be quiet!" Instead of telling the whole group to be quiet, I was singled out as the only child making noise. I did not notice this, as I was always singled out for special attention, but it was very noticeable to my mother and all the other parents who had come to see their little darlings participate in the show.

The final straw came a few days later. As part of the Australian theme, the children had to dress up in period costume.

I went as the famous Australian bushranger, Ned Kelly, who fascinated me at the time. A relative had made an excellent replica of Ned Kelly's metal armor. First, on went the chest armor. Next was a brown all-weather trench coat, complete with bloody bandages painted with red lipstick to represent his wounds when shot by the troopers. Finally, on went the familiar Kelly helmet complete with an eye slit opening and a pistol in each hand. I really looked the part. My father delivered me to school and observed what happened. I was late and everyone was already in class. When I walked into the room the class

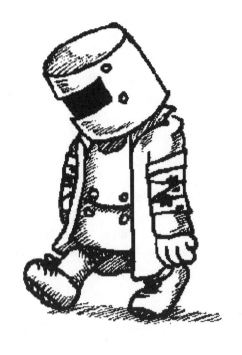

erupted, clapping and cheering. They knew it was me because I was the only one missing from the class roll call. The teacher barely moved, just looked up from his desk, told the class to be quiet and told me to take off my ridiculous costume, put it at the back of the room and sit down at my desk. What a let down! I was admired by the class but put down again by another teacher.

My father was watching this through the glass windows in the corridor. Furiously, he stormed out of the school and told my mother what had happened. To my parents it was obvious I had been labeled by the teachers. I was not going to get a fair go. I was about to leave my first school after only six months.

But now I don't really care any more. What's done is done, I guess. Anyway, I hated school in my early days. I was not stupid. I just couldn't concentrate like other kids, which affected my behavior and my learning ability. I would go to school crying, cry at school and then come home crying. It was not that I was a crybaby and liked crying. It was, I guess, that I never knew exactly why I was in trouble. To the teachers I was just a bad kid who disrupted the class too often. Schools are not made for children like me. But the problem is that we have to go to school and we will never be able to change that. But schools can and should recognize the problems of an ADD child. Passing problem students such as me on and on to another school resolves nothing. It only causes more problems for such students. They often leave school when they are old enough without completing their studies. This makes me sad because if I had left school prematurely, as many ADD children do, I would not have the academic grounding I do today— and this book would not have been written.

It makes me laugh to look back on my report cards now. Nothing really changed from prep to Year Twelve. They all go like this:

> Benjamin has the ability to do better but needs to focus more of his extensive energy into doing more useful and productive things. He lacks good concentration skills and has trouble listening to instructions. He often involves himself in inappropriate activity such as entertaining the class by being the center of attention.

In my early days, language skills and mathematics were often cause for concern. My sporting abilities were always excellent and it was something I enjoyed. Sport is a great way for children with ADD to burn off excess energy. I still use exercise as a tool to help me settle down. Sport also gives these children a chance to build self-esteem, which is often hard to achieve in the classroom. Lack of self-esteem was a problem that I had to overcome in my early years. This age is crucial for children. It is when they learn essential interpersonal skills. This period can be the time when a child's feelings towards school can be made or destroyed. Well, my feelings towards school developed pretty soon. I hated it!

In the classroom, impulsiveness and standing out are a bad mixture. The problem arises due to low self-esteem. ADD children often fall behind in schoolwork, receive the unwanted attention of the teacher, become separated and suffer from low self-esteem. The ADD child is constantly being made to feel different from the rest of the kids. The ADD child wants to be "normal" but does not understand why he is not. They look the same but just don't seem to fit in with the rest of the children. Other children often use an ADD child as a scapegoat. When the ADD child is told to do something by the other kids he goes at it like a bull at a gate. This is caused by impulsiveness—not thinking before acting. As a parent, you must learn to build self-esteem in your child. This topic will be discussed in later chapters.

My problem was that I loved being the center of attention and would usually do the most foolish things just to get a laugh. This is why I was in so much trouble when I was young. Now I understand and realize that the other kids were just using me as a bit of a joke.

I spent most of my early school days sitting in the punishment corner wondering what was wrong with me. My parents remember me dressed in my school uniform crying, every day pleading for my parents to let me stay home. Something had to change and it did. They rationalized that maybe a private school with smaller classes would help. Well, off to a private school I went, tie and all!

Private school – Year 1 to Year 4

The private school was expensive, and had smaller classes, but for me nothing changed, except that the teachers could spend more time with individual students.

GRADE ONE REPORT CARD:

Expression	Achievement	
Listening skills	B	Ben's oral expression is clear and confident
Oral expression	B	and his written expression has shown great
Written expression	C	improvement. Ben generally makes an effort
		to listen attentively

Reading	Achievement	
Oral reading	C	Ben tries hard in reading and is developing
Comprehension	B	quite well. He enjoys books and makes good
Word Attack Skills	C	use of the class and school library.

Spelling	Achievement	
Spells assigned words	B	Ben has worked very hard to develop his
Applies spelling		spelling skills with very good results, both in
Skills in writing	B	written work and with set words.

Handwriting	Achievement	
Letter formation	B	Ben's handwriting is quite fluent with good
Fluency	B	letter formation when he takes the time to
Bookwork/		write carefully.
Organization	Not shown	

Physical Education	Achievement	
Motor Skills	A	Ben is very aggressive towards his sport. He
		is a coordinated and confident student.
Participation	B	Ben is still learning tolerance towards those
		who do not perform as well as he does. He is
		making progress in this regard.

Social behavior and learning skills

Respects the rights of others	Not seen yet
Accepts constructive criticism	Excellent
Participates actively	Excellent
Courteous in speech and manner	Not seen yet
Relates well	Not seen yet
Begins work promptly	Not seen yet
Concentrates on tasks	Excellent
Shares duties willingly	Excellent
Helps others in need	Not seen yet
Organizes own belongings	Not seen yet

The report looks good but in my opinion it's not true. I couldn't do the work that most of the children could. I could not read, spell or write and I did not enjoy books. I was very below standard in all areas except sports. I could not read the most basic words or complete basic math. The conclusion I have drawn from this is that the new school was not going to tell my parents that I was academically not up to standard compared to the other students, especially when parents are paying thousands of dollars a year.

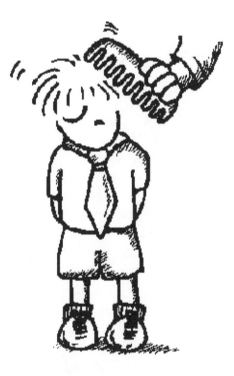

Academically, I was pretty unsuccessful. This problem often arises with ADD children. They are not stupid, often quite bright. But they learn in totally different ways to other children. The only problem is that ADD children usually must learn in the conventional manner. To overcome this, many parents employ remedial tutors or do a lot of the teaching one-on-one with their child. This is a difficult period for both the parents and the child. The child must learn to read and write or face falling behind in school and subsequently in life.

Here are the major problems. The child does not have the same attention span as other children and loses interest very quickly. Homework is often an issue that ends in tears, yelling and sometimes violent conflict. The child falls further and further behind until he is so far below the other children that he believes he is truly stupid.

The ADD child is often seen as a daydreamer in class. This is because other more exciting thoughts are going on inside their heads. It is a very challenging time for both teachers and parents. Unfortunately, there is no easy answer. As a parent, you must persist until your child can read and write at a level that will allow them to progress to higher classes. ADD children often repeat grades in their early years. I strongly disagree with this policy because it contributes to a major problem—low self-esteem. The ADD child already feels different, isolated and stupid. Leaving them behind just reinforces this belief.

I am currently tutoring a boy who told me, "The other kids don't have to do this extra work." I replied, "You're right, the kids don't have to do this work because they have already done it a couple of years ago." We had a little talk about this. I tried to explain to him that everyone has to learn to read and that it takes time. I told him that he had been wasting his time by mucking around and not doing his homework. I asked him, "Do you want to read?" He replied, "Yes." "What's stopping you then?" He replied, "Nothing, I guess." "That's not true. You are stopping yourself. Why?" His answer, "I don't know." I then asked him again, "Do you want to read?" Again he replied, "Yes, I told you that."

Making him think to himself, 'Why can't I read like the other kids?' made crucial progress in this situation. Once he realized that he himself was the reason he could not read, his effort increased dramatically and so did his results.

When using this technique of trying to make your child accept responsibility for their lack of progress in something, you must pick your words very carefully. You are in danger of causing the child's already low self-esteem to be further damaged. You must make the child feel that he can do anything that he can put his mind to. Once they achieve something they had thought they could not do, you can use this achievement to reinforce a positive thought process.

This technique comes from my own personal experiences. My father always told me, "You can do it!" At the age of five I could snow ski better than most adults. My father taught me by holding me between his legs and then letting me go so I had to ski by myself. I would crash and start crying. "Get up!" my father would say. Then we would do it all over again. Every time I fell over I would get up and do it all again. I became so good my father took me down the hardest runs, mostly on my backside. When we got to the bottom he would tell me that I had just completed a black run (the hardest run). The next time he told me we were going down a black run and I didn't want to go, he would say, "You have done it before, did you get hurt?" I would reply, "No." "So what's stopping you? Let's go!"

Because I thought I could do anything, my confidence skyrocketed. I became so good I would ski around adults who had fallen over, spray snow all over them and yell out, "Suffer!" This occurred so often my father would punish me because during the long wait for the next chairlift he would see adults glaring at the father with the nasty ski whiz kid. But I still kept on doing it! It was too much fun to miss out on!

You must find something, anything, that your child is good at, to build self-esteem. Sport is extremely useful for all children at this age, but especially for ADD children. When competing at sport their unlimited supply of energy and eagerness often shines brightly. I believe individual sports are best for young ADD children. They are often isolated in team sports due to their behavior. Individual sports create excellent self-esteem because they find they did it all by themselves. It also allows these children an outlet to let off steam, instead of releasing their anger and frustration on their parents. ADD children often get bored doing the same thing, so when this happens you need to be prepared to change or to try another sport. Most importantly, try to get your child to pick the next sport. This makes them responsible for their actions and avoids the problem when they say to their mum or dad, "It's your fault, Mum. You made me do this!" This idea of encouragement and trying to create a positive mental attitude is not a new concept but it is a crucial tactic for any parent trying to overcome low self-esteem in their child, particularly in the early-school years.

Grade Two!

At this time I continued to struggle with both schoolwork and behavior. I was improving with reading and writing, but was still below average. My teacher at the time was Mrs. Yates. I would like to say thank you to this lovely person who had the patience and cared enough to help me to learn how to read. Without her, this would not have been possible. It was Mrs. Yates who recognized my reading and spelling problems and instigated a reading-recovery program. Every day after school I would stay back with her and learn the basics of reading. During this period I truly thought I was just *stupid!* I remember one occasion as if it were yesterday. She asked me to spell "of" and I sounded out the word and spelt it "ov"—the way it sounds. It was obviously wrong and I couldn't believe how dumb I was in not spelling a basic two-letter word correctly. It's words like this that makes learning the English language so hard and frustrating. It's difficult trying to explain to a child that they must remember and then learn how to use words, but that not all words can be simply sounded out. This is especially difficult when teaching an ADD student. Short-term memory

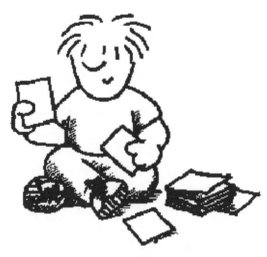

problems are common with ADD students and magnify the difficulty in remembering difficult words, such as "of," commonly found in the English language.

Mrs. Yates and I persisted every day after school, then again with my parents at home. I hated reading and still hate forced reading today, such as massive university books. The problem is not with the reading itself or the content of the book. Children with ADD don't have the concentration and patience to continue reading when it gets boring for them so quickly. To tell the truth, I read my first book from cover to cover only a couple of months ago. Maybe you find that hard to believe, but it is true. I think it is quite amusing and some people may think it is impossible that a 19-year-old university student who completely read his first book only a couple of months ago is now writing his own.

While reading my first book ever I wondered how I could keep interested and concentrate on one topic for hours on end. I thought about this a lot and then it hit me—I wasn't reading the book as I had used to do. I was a part of the book. Instead of reading just words, I was visualizing what the words were describing and saying. This was a real breakthrough for me and I will describe later how you can use this technique with your own child's education. It really works wonders. I hated reading anything at school. I didn't even read my three novels in Year Twelve English and that was my second highest study score in my overall score. My mother even went to extraordinary lengths to help me read my year Twelve English novels. She rang up the Blind Society and got them on tape for me. But I didn't use them. However, I did lend them to my friends at school and they found them very useful. When they gave them back to me, I lost some of the taped books. The Blind Society rang me to get them back and I didn't have the courage to tell them that I had lost them. So I used my quick-thinking ADD brain and told the lady, "I am blind and I can't see them or find them!" She had pity on me and I felt so bad!

To overcome this problem, you must find out what your child is interested in and use it to your advantage. My parents did this by using Teenage Mutant Ninja Turtles trading cards (a craze with children at the time). I was obsessed with these cards. Because they had only a little bit of information on the back of the card I could focus enough to read the back of these cards every night, because they interested me. This is where you can use your child's short attention span to good use.

As my academic skills improved, my confidence again increased. Once your child has mastered the basic words they should progress at an alarming speed. This is because they are not stupid, they just learn differently. I will discuss techniques in the later chapters that show you how to tap into your child's interests and capture that elusive attention span. This may seem strange but I can study for 12 hours straight (without medication) using the self-help techniques I have developed.

This is the comment from my teacher in Grade Two:

> Ben is a pleasant, reliable member of the class. He is always
> ready to help someone in trouble. The improvement he is
> making in reading and spelling is giving him a great boost
> in confidence, which is very good to see. I hope this
> continues in the second half of the year.
>
> Mrs. Yates

With a lot of hard work my academic progress improved greatly. But my behavior was still an issue. One day our class went outside to play a game, I don't remember exactly what it was. A girl was doing handstands in the sports shed while we were waiting for the teacher. I joined in and also did a handstand. She pushed me over and I fell. Well, I was so angry at her that when she did another handstand I pushed her over with extreme force. This is a common reaction of an ADD child. They don't think about the consequences of their actions. They just act. She fell over and started crying. I was sent to the principal's office without any explanation and without being able to give my side of the story. Situations like this happened often. The ADD child is always the one who gets in trouble when in his mind he has done nothing wrong. This creates a lot of confusion and greatly upsets him because he does not understand why he is always getting into trouble. I was outside the principal's office, waiting to be blasted again, I thought to myself, "Well, I'm not wanted here," so I took off and ran away from school.

The school was on a long road with farmlets on both sides. I ran up the road with the school principal in hot pursuit in the school bus. It would have looked pretty amusing for anyone driving past. I was caught, taken back to school and got into even more trouble. I hated school again! I had to go back but this time the older kids thought I was a legend. From that day on I was known as the kid who had run away from school.

Grade Three!

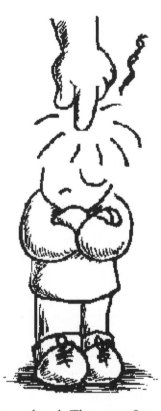

Nothing much changed except that I had a new teacher who could not handle me and I couldn't handle her. She hated me and I hated her. We had a personality conflict. She was a strong feminist, who didn't like hyperactive, rude and opinionated students like me. She was straight out of teachers' college and not ready for a boy like me. She would make me feel stupid, highlighting my mistakes to the class and always pointing her finger at me. The girls in the class were her favorites and they knew it. They would blame me for everything that went wrong in her class. These girls and I have spoken about her since, and they still laugh when they tell me how they got away with everything by using me as the scapegoat. As a consequence of my ill treatment, my anger and behavior problems at home escalated. The more I got into trouble at school the more confused I became. This would then flow on to my home life. I constantly hit my sister, the dog, anybody and anything, just to release my anger. I was out of control. I knew it and my parents knew it. I know that I was out of control because I contemplated suicide because I hated myself so much and I didn't know why.

Grade Four!

Well, I got that teacher again. I feel this should not be allowed because it is extremely unfair for children who do not like a teacher, because their studies will be affected. I fell further and further behind in class and my parents became extremely worried. It was during this time the principal recommended I see a child psychiatrist. This is the report written by the psychiatrist to my parents.

CONFIDENTIAL PSYCHOLOGICAL REPORT
NAME: BEN POLIS
REFERRED BY: PRINCIPAL OF COLLEGE
Ben presented as an energetic eight-year-old child who attends local private college. He has a ten-year-old sister (Adelaide) who attends a primary school. Mr. Polis was concerned at Ben's behavior and seemed extremely willing to gain help for himself and family as well as for Ben, to understand and learn how to control Ben's behavior.

Mr Polis told me that Adelaide was very socially accepted and usually exhibited excellent behavior, but Ben, although happy, was causing problems at home and, to a lesser extent, at school because of his behavior. Ben suffers from asthma and has previously seen a child psychiatrist.

I saw Ben on four occasions and spoke with Mr. Polis on each of these. I spoke with Adelaide on one occasion. Mrs. Polis did not attend any sessions. It is my opinion that Ben's behavior signifies an attention deficit disorder with hyperactivity. Ben's behaviors include inattentiveness, impulsivity, aggression and disobedience.

When dealing with a child who exhibits this type of behavior parents need to be aware of the following: While a "normal" child might not want to do something, the hyperactive child will refuse point blank and have a tantrum if pressed. The child has trouble remembering instructions, a firm *"No"* is forgotten within hours.

Because his brain becomes intensely over stimulated by any mental exertion, instructions of any kind tend to evoke a wild and uncontrolled response. Be prepared to repeat many, many more times all the edicts and instructions the "normal" child learns and remembers quite quickly.

Most hyperactive children do not respond to voice alone. This is not deliberately ignoring the parent, but because they do not process incoming information in the normal way. Even the sound of their own name, repeated several times, may not get a response. Try touching the child to attract attention.

Get him to look at you and focus his attention on you before you speak. Shouting at him will produce more confusion in his brain and may make him have a tantrum. If this child's confidence in his parents is undermined by mixed messages it magnifies the problem, therefore it is extremely important that he receive consistent messages from both parents about behavior and how they feel about him as a person.

There is growing evidence that allergies can cause hyperactivity in a susceptible child. The children may be allergically sensitive to foods and also sensitive to inhaled allergens. Ben and his family need to be aware, because of his asthma and hyperactivity, of his food intake (diet) and inhalants. Ben needs to be disciplined in this area. He needs a lot of positive reinforcement when he is behaving well and often needs things explained more than other children need to have. His food intake needs to be monitored to see what foods cause his behavior to increase or stabilize.

If there are any further issues you would like to discuss with me, I will be happy to do so.

Searching through my extensive medical records and finding this report was a surprise to my parents because we thought I was diagnosed at 12 years old, but it clearly states that I was diagnosed when I was 8 years old. The problem was that ADD was not readily recognized and treated as it is today, especially in

Victoria, Australia. We were very behind in the diagnosis of ADD compared to the other states. This has changed substantially today with ADD becoming better recognized not only in Victoria but also world-wide. The psychologist recommended better parenting techniques and modifying my diet. Unfortunately this was not the solution. Due to

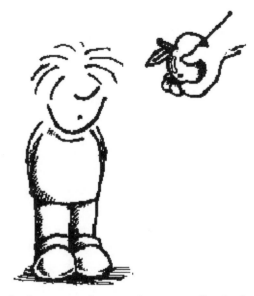

my allergic reactions to foods that caused my asthma my diet had always been modified. I was never placed on a controlled diet for my ADD. But I have a problem believing that diet could greatly change the psychological make-up of one's brain. Studies state that only 5 per cent of subjects studied have shown any improvement. I have no doubt that modified diets could reduce hyperactivity because we have all seen what happens sometimes when kids drink too much red cordial. But I am still very skeptical. My parents were good parents and strictly controlled my behavior. We found out later I simply needed medication to increase my concentration and learning retention. Before we go on, please let me state firmly that I do not believe that medication by itself is the solution to modifying a child's ADD behavior. Medication is not the answer to ADD and never will be! Your child must learn to control their behavior, learn to adjust and modify the way they act. And parents who love your child, you must help and show them how. I could concentrate when I had to. I could do the work when I had to and I could behave well when I wanted to. But I didn't then, because I simply did not know how to turn on my concentration and modify my behavior, as I do now.

Little boys should not play with big boys' toys

It was the Easter holiday in 1990 and five families went to Cape Paterson, a Victorian seaside holiday resort township, to surf, fish and just relax. Not this year though, for Benjamin Polis had arrived. We stayed in the local caravan park facing the roaring ocean of Bass Strait. My father and his friend were keen skindivers, snorkeling for fish with a spear gun or a Hawaiian sling, a spear about two meters long with barbed points at one end and a strong elastic rubber band at the other end which fires the spear at the fish. I was only nine years old but, boy, do I remember this incident. My father and his mate came back from skindiving and left their spears at the front of the caravan. I grabbed my dad's Hawaiian sling to show cousin Lachlan how it worked, shooting it vertically about ten meters high into the air. I repeated this a number of times, until a strong gust of wind blew the spear onto the power lines. It created a short circuit between the two wires. This happened all in a blink of an eye. The power pole that Lachlan and I were standing under exploded with sparks flying everywhere. It looked like a bad day in Bosnia. The current then flowed through all the other poles, blowing them up one after the other in a big circle around the caravan park. Every power line connected between the poles fell to the ground, just missing tents and caravans. People came running to see what had happened. I don't know how it was that no one was killed or injured. The only wires that did not fall were the two with

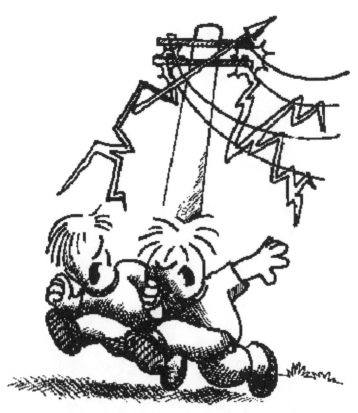

the aluminium spear still lying across them. A State Electricity Commission team arrived to repair the damage.

I did not see any of this because I hid in the caravan for hours in my bunk, covered with sleeping bags. Frightened like any other child, I thought that what I could not see could not hurt me. I remember thinking to myself, "I can't do anything right." Even now, thinking back, this was a period in my life that still makes me upset. I wanted to die and even contemplated killing myself. This seems pretty sad when you remember that I was only nine, but I lived through this nightmare over and over when I was younger. I was different, stupid, always in trouble and everyone hated me. Well, that's not true, but that's what I thought at the time.

Dad told me that after the repair team worked most of the day repairing the lines, the foreman asked some people, which included Dad, about the incident. The foreman asked, "Do you know who did this? Now, before you answer I am telling you the repair bill for the damage is around $13,000 and if the parents of the boy who did this had any sense they would pack up immediately and leave the park. Do you know what I mean?" My father may be honest, but he is not stupid. And that's what we did and we have never gone back to Cape Paterson since. I would just like to thank the man who told my dad that we had to leave because otherwise I would still be paying it back today.

The above is an example of when an ADD child does something without realizing the consequences of their actions. I could not foresee that playing with a spear near power lines could result in so much damage and possibly kill someone. My parents were upset but I was not punished in any way. It was bad enough that I was punishing myself. I could understand being punished by my parents but what would that have achieved? More important was my mental condition. Feeling stupid, always getting into trouble, I needed support, not more punishment. Fortunately that's what I got from my parents and that is my advice to other parents. Don't punish a child who is already down. No matter how hard it is to give at times, you must give your child that support, particularly at the worst of times. If you punish them and give no support when they are fragile and vulnerable, who will support them when they need it the most?

Let's now consider another situation where two ADD symptoms combine—impulsiveness with determination/stubbornness. This experience was written in Year Twelve for a VCE English writing assignment. It was meant to be a creative writing exercise, but the story is true, like everything else in this book.

He who dares wins!

As I look back on my childhood there is one significant experience I remember that sticks in my mind as vividly as the night it all unfolded. It was around four o'clock when my family and I set off from our caravan that was on land adjacent to a national park. The national park was about thirty kilometres from the heart of Sydney. As we set off on the walking trail it seemed to be engulfed by a veranda of vines and scrub that encircled us as we walked further and further into the unknown. As we were walking, it seems somewhat foolish now looking back on it, but the family was more interested in our conversation than where we were walking.

As the day passed and dusk set in, the night sky darkened with every step and the conversation intensified. I began to question my parents about what might be lurking in the thick scrub. The scrub was now only a vision of dark shadows that seemed to join with the night sky. "Scared, Ben?" Dad asked. I replied, "No." But I was only ten and truly was scared of the dark and especially the uncertainty of the moment. My parents and my older sister, Adelaide, began to tease and taunt me about the fictional "Boogie Man" that I believed in. I was continually being asked "Is that the Boogie Man, Ben? Oooooo!" I fell behind, and they let me continue alone along the path. My mother then dared me to walk back to the caravan by myself, for one hundred dollars. This was a lot of money at the time for a ten-year-old. After a couple of minutes of weighing up the pros and cons, being a mad Ninja Turtles fan at the time swayed my decision. Thinking to myself of how many new figurines I could buy with the money, I set off by myself to the caravan to win and claim my prize.

I thought to myself that the quickest and most accurate way to get home was to walk straight ahead and follow the lights twinkling

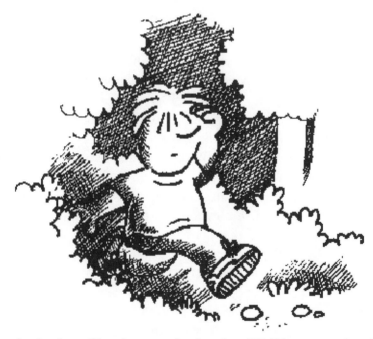

on the horizon like the stars in the sky. Walking soon developed into a fast jog, trying not to think of the Boogie Man that every few seconds flashed through my mind like a recurring nightmare. Running, I focused my entire attention straight ahead on the Ninja Turtles that I could buy, if only I made it.

Meanwhile, my parents thought that I would turn around and find them. They planned that when I did they would all jump out and scare the hell out of me. The only problem with this plan was they did not believe that I would walk home. After realizing that I was not coming after them, they ran around frantically searching. By this time I had made it and started to wonder where my family was. To kill time, I took some money from my mum's handbag that I intended to pay back with my one hundred dollars, which I was beginning to long for. I set off to play video games in the caravan park's game room.

My parents by this stage had got themselves lost and finally made their way to a ranger's house in the national park. Well, the ranger got on the horn to his mates and within fifteen minutes they had six rangers searching and scouring the bush, now totally immersed by the cover of darkness. A couple of hours later, sitting in the caravan because the games room had closed, I started to panic. "Where is my family?" Many hours later they turned up to find me in my bunk fast asleep.

This experience shows my early determination to succeed when pushed hard enough by myself. This is something that I must do every day because I can be very lazy when I do not force myself. For example, writing this book. Like a lot of things, it frustrates me and I give up easily when things get too hard or boring. However, I force myself to do things by shutting myself off from everyone. Sometimes I feel a bit like the Dalai Lama, putting myself in self-imposed exile.

Grade Five and off to another school!

It was the first day of Grade Five at the private school with a new teacher. He was a good teacher and all the children loved him. He was a tough but fair man—just what I needed. My parents and I thought it was good for me to have a male teacher who would be able to handle my boisterous behavior, especially since I had usually had female teachers since prep.

Things were looking good for me. However, the hatred of my previous teacher still burned like a wild fire, so I did something incredibly stupid. I wanted to pay her back for the way she had treated me for the past two years. Someone was passing around a magazine with a cartoon of two people having sex. So I thought,

"Right, I'll get her this time!" Firstly, I wrote the name of her boyfriend on the man's head. He was on top of the woman. Then I wrote her name on the woman's head. I put a talking bubble coming from my ex-teacher's mouth with the words, "Ooo Baby!" and then stuck it in the teacher's diary so that when she opened it up the following day she would have a pleasant surprise. Well, I guess she did because I got kicked out the next day!

That was a rude shock to me because I never thought I would be expelled from school. Well, I was wrong and it was the first of many schools that would use the big E word on me. My parents were not pleased at me getting kicked out. However, it did improve their cash flow. Dad rang the nearest government primary school and told them they had a new student. There was some objection because the school was already full. By this stage, I think my father had had enough. He told the principal something along the lines that the law required his son to be educated, this was the nearest government school and this was where he would be going.

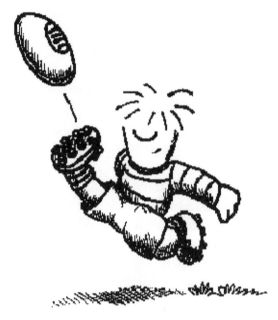

My new primary was a good school and I had a teacher who could really handle me. He made me hate him because he was just like me and challenged me in every way. I was always trying to show him up by being a big shot and class clown. I have always had a problem with authority and still do. I don't care who someone is or what position they hold, it does not matter to me. I treat people who deserve to be respected with respect, but if I feel they do not deserve respect from me, they get none. This would get me into trouble at school and at work when I was older. This teacher was always throwing me out of class when I cracked a joke or was just being myself, which was being a typical ADD kid. The problem was in my mind—he did not practice what he preached. If he could crack jokes all the time, why couldn't I? Because he was the teacher and I was the student. But I couldn't see that because of my lack of respect for authority.

During Grade Five I spent many weeks in the Children's Hospital again with asthma. I still have many get-well cards from students and teachers, and it makes me laugh when I read them. I cherish the card that my Grade Five classmates gave me because it is so true and pretty funny. The card goes something like this:

GET WELL SOON

To Dear Ben,
It gets a bit quiet in the classroom when you're not here and I've got no one to pick on. So get well quick and get back here!
From your teacher

THE STUDENTS' COMMENTS:
To Ben, it's not funny at school any more!
Get back here, it's boring without 'cha!
To Ben, you don't annoy us any more!
To Ben, I hope you get well soon.
P.S. I hope you come back so I can see you get into trouble!

Grade Five saw my academic progress improve substantially. I believe that the primary school was good for me because the children came from average families. This made it easier to interact with the other kids. The primary kids played sports at lunchtime and were a lot more boisterous. This was great for me or any ADD child who has excess energy to burn. I started to take up Australian Rules football, again giving me another avenue to release my anger and frustration rather than directing it at my parents and teachers. My school report had the following comments:

ENGLISH:
A great improvement in attitude towards language work in general has allowed Ben to achieve a lot this year.

MATHEMATICS:
Has the potential to do well when he puts his mind to it. Ben displays the skills necessary to produce results.

GENERAL STUDIES:
A big effort is needed to be a co-operative member of a group. Occasionally he shows he possesses excellent knowledge and skills.

ART:
Ben has good artistic skills but tends not to display them due to a lack of concentration.

GENERAL COMMENTS:
Ben has shown great improvement in his attitude towards his work. With a greater effort to stay on task and not enter into every conversation in the classroom without thinking about the consequences of his actions, his work will improve even more. Ben also needs to show a little more compassion towards the other children and not attempt to talk over them all the time.

Grade Six!

During Grade Six my behavior became worse, and I was constantly assaulting students, my parents and sister. Homework was always a problem and this was a serious concern for my parents because I was just about to enter high school. I had joined a basketball team and assaulted one of my team mates because he was annoying me. Incidents like this were regular during the year. Neither my parents nor teachers could control me any more. I was growing up and fast. I did what I wanted, when I wanted.

This school, like all my schools, had finally had enough of me, especially my art teacher. Children with ADD can do well in these subjects if they have artistic flair. Art has never been one of my strong points. Like a lot of ADD children, the problem I have in these types of subjects is that the unstructured classroom set-up is often too overwhelming. The problem with subjects such as woodwork, textiles and art is that they often need a high level of concentration to stay on task. To try to get an ADD child to paint a picture on his own is nearly impossible. An ADD child is often distracted by all the paints and tools in these classrooms. Eating the paint or painting the kid next to him is often more appealing in these subjects. This is not the case in all situations. An ADD child can do well if they really enjoy the subject.

However, I did not enjoy them. Well, that's not true: I did enjoy the subjects because they were so much fun—I could get up to so much mischief. On an academic scale I did not do well. An example of this was Year Eleven woodwork. I did this subject because it was a breeze. Well, I thought it would be a breeze. I have good manual skills and this comes from my father teaching me over and over again how to use tools in the shed. I have restored furniture and built things. He always tried so hard to teach me to use every tool and when I didn't use them properly he would be very angry with me.

Anyway, I nearly failed woodwork in Year Eleven. It was not that I couldn't do the work, it was that I could not stay on task. I was more interested in talking and just having fun. Also, these subjects are usually at the end of the day in a double period. An ADD child by the end of the day can hardly concentrate enough to tie his shoelaces. This is a huge problem. You place an ADD child in a class like this at the end of the day when his concentration is at its lowest point to work independently on a task in a classroom full of distraction? It ain't going to happen! This is a recipe for disaster.

This was very true in Grade Six. Visualize the following situation. It was the last twenty minutes on a Friday after a long week and I was not at my best. I was tired, frustrated and mentally bored in class. I had to make something out of clay fast. I had been fooling around rolling out a 45cm penis. I then had a brainwave, "Let's make a face that looks like a penis." Very amusing for an ADD child and the other students. I cleverly molded the clay into shape. The penis at first looked like a nose, but then was readily

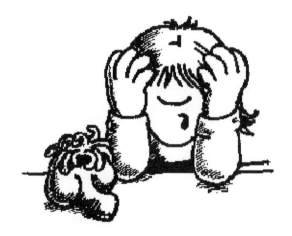

recognizable as a penis, with eyes that looked like testicles and added hair which resembled pubic hair. I just finished my masterpiece in the nick of time. I placed the masterpiece on the teacher's desk so she could put it in the kiln. Did she like my masterpiece? No, she nearly died! The following Monday my father and I were summoned to see the principal and art teacher. I remember this so clearly, I thought it was so funny. My art teacher said calmly and politely, "Benjamin made a very large male anatomy!" I denied it for about ten minutes. "It's a face! I don't see what's wrong with it, I like it!" Anyway, they wanted to expel me but again my dad pleaded for me to stay.

My parents and teachers soon observed a pattern in my behavior. I would constantly be in trouble, usually in the afternoon, because I was tired and bored. This pattern continued into my high-school years. What I am trying to say is that if you can prevent your ADD child from having these types of classes in the afternoon it will be beneficial for both you and the school. Unfortunately in primary school you have little control over timetables. In high school you can choose your subjects to a certain degree. Irrespective of timetables, you need to be prepared for trouble in afternoon classes and explain to the school why it happens. It is also worth noting that stimulant medication often wears off in the afternoon, only adding to the problem.

Every day I would furiously ride my bike out of the school and do a big burnout in front of all the parents waiting to pick up their children. Many parents hated me and gave me glares and stares. I loved this and would deliberately pick on their children. It was a big game to me and I loved the attention. There was a common belief I acted in such a manner because I was a spoiled brat, because my parents were well off. This impression followed me everywhere I went. I always had the newest brand-name shoes and clothes and would rub it in to others. I am so competitive in everything I do and I hate to lose. This may be due to the low self-esteem I had when I was younger. Other children would be friends until they came to our house, and saw that I had lots of toys and so on. Then they would ignore me at school.

This also happened at sports clubs. When I was eleven I joined the local cricket club and my dad bought me all the new gear as soon as I started. The other kids were so jealous they picked on me and would push me around. One Saturday I ran off from the cricket ground where we were playing. I walked home, and it took me hours. Schools and sports clubs—I changed them often because I would wear out my welcome. Eventually, this was resolved by taking me out of our area to play cricket in a wealthier suburb. I still can't understand why people reacted this way—it was not my fault my parents could afford to buy things. What's the point of working hard and being successful, if you can't enjoy the extra money by spending it on your children?

You may be thinking that I deserved this treatment because I would boast about having all these great things. But this did not happen until I was much older. I turned it into a game. If people were going to be jealous of me because I had new clothes all the time I could not do anything about it. I was not going to take back the new clothes my parents had bought me, was I? So instead I turned it around and sought enjoyment by deliberately showing off my new things. They were going to dislike me anyway so I just made them hate me even more. It was more fun that way.

Because of my bad behavior everyone in the area knew me, for the wrong reasons. A real-estate agent must cultivate a good reputation to get work in his area of operations or "look after his vegetable patch" as dad would say. I was such a monster they believed people would not want to use my father as their agent. My parents thought I was bad for their business. To overcome my bad name in the area (after three schools and three sports clubs) I started going to schools further and further away. My parents always joked I would end up in Darwin because I had worn out my welcome in Victoria. They also discussed sending me to a boarding school in Darwin because I would not be able to run home as I could and did in Melbourne. They were only joking—I think.

My diagnosis of ADHD!

During Year Seven my behavior became so bad my mother could not handle me any more. She was determined to find out what was wrong with her son. She had already taken me to many child psychiatrists with no solutions except for them suggesting better parenting techniques. In desperation, she contacted the Royal Children's Hospital, the same place that had saved my life in 1984 when I was in intensive care with chronic asthma. Her initial contact was a senior physician at the Centre for Adolescent Health, who was not an expert on ADD but who referred me to another child psychiatrist. This time we were getting somewhere. Every week for months, we went to the Children's Hospital to see my new doctor. At first I didn't like going because he would ask probing personal questions but at the same time he understood me a lot better than anyone had before. He placed me on stimulants—methylphenidate, or Ritalin. My behavior did not change immediately, in fact it didn't change much for about three to four years. I guess this is really what this book is all about.

I have ADHD and I had to learn to live with it. I had to learn to modify my behavior and retrain the way my brain works. Medications help but they will not resolve my impulsiveness, anger, low concentration and frantic bursts of activity followed by long periods of laziness. I had to learn how to control myself because I couldn't keep taking Ritalin all the time to modify my behavior. I would rather be unmedicated for the rest of my life than be medicated day in day out. Most parents and doctors don't really understand how it feels to be knocked out by this

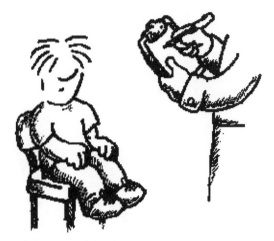

medication for days on end. Doctors believe that it is perfectly safe to be on this medication for long periods of time and I am sure it is. But have there been any studies done on the mental strain of having a hyper-stimulated thought process for months and even years on end? These drugs work best when you use them in moderation. What I mean by this is that you should use them only when you need to. What is the point of medicating your child if he sits there just watching television in an unnatural zombie state?

This is the letter my doctor wrote to the physician to thank him for referring me as a patient.

4th June 1994

Thank you for referring the above named. I saw Benjamin Polis with his parents on two occasions. Benjamin has a long history of behavior problems. At present there is severe family disharmony because of Ben's behavior. The parents felt they could no longer cope.

When reviewing the history, there was good evidence that Benjamin suffers from Attention Deficit Hyperactivity Disorder. At present, the main difficulty is his impulsiveness.

During an individual interview, Benjamin was cooperative. He was fidgety. No evidence of anxiety or depressive disorder. He felt very negative towards his father but was willing to cooperate with treatment.

I have started cognitive behavioral therapy to help Ben. Because of the urgency of this situation, I think combining the use of stimulant medication is justified. The parents and Ben are happy with this after discussion. I will start him on low doses of methylphenidate and will continue to see him on an outpatient basis.

Year Seven at Secondary college

My sister made the decision for me to be sent to a different Secondary college than hers. She was embarrassed to have me as her brother and did not want to have any social contact with me. I do not blame her for this because I did not have the best reputation in the area. My name did and still does follow me everywhere I go today, but I do not mind this. In fact, I get a real kick out of telling people what I am doing now, to see their faces change when I tell them I'm at university. Whenever people ask, "Whatever happened to that wild son of yours?" both my parents have great pride in telling people who had labeled me a loser all those years ago that I am at university. My mother also finds it quite funny when mothers ask her what I am doing and she tells them. But for some reason they never tell her what their son is doing! Funny about that!

Year Seven was most probably the worst year of my life. Once again I hated the school and the school hated me. This was the first time I started to feel totally embarrassed about having Attention Deficit Hyperactivity Disorder. My mother told the school of my medical condition, hopefully to get a little bit of understanding

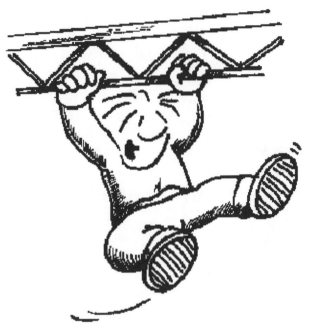

when I played up. I openly admit that in Year Seven I was completely out of control. Failing every subject with flying colors!

Looking back on it now, I believe there is a good reason for my behavior and dismal academic record. In primary school, everything was in a repetitive format. Being told when to sit and when to stand up is perfect for a child like me. However, at secondary school this routine that was easy to comply with and understand was gone. I had to organize myself to get up in time and catch a train and a bus. When I did finally get to school (usually late) I then had to get my books and find my class. Unlike the stability of a primary school, you change classrooms every period. I would forget books, homework, sports clothes and so on and continually draw unwanted attention to myself because I was totally disorganized. This is why I believe that if your child does have ADD you must train your child in primary school to learn to become more independent, better organized at school and home, and to take care of themselves. If you do not, they will be overwhelmed by the lack of routine in secondary school and their academic progress and behavior will suffer.

This is exactly what happened to me. One day in a French class we were doing a test and I couldn't answer even the first question. I sat there thinking, "I am so dumb!" After five minutes of just sitting, boredom set in. Like any other ADD child, I started to amuse myself by annoying the person next to me, then the teacher. I asked if I could shut the windows because it was cold, which it was not, but I was amusing myself. I climbed up onto the window sill to shut the top window. Everyone was looking at me and I love an audience. So I pretended to fall! As I was falling, I grabbed the roof rafter and swung back and forwards a couple of times. I then impulsively pretended to fall again, but this time I was not pretending. I fell and accidentally kicked a boy in the head. In trouble again! The teacher yelled at the top of her lungs, "Go to C3!"—the time-out room when you are removed from class.

I don't know why they didn't just send me there and leave me there because I spent most of the year there. In the past couple of years I have spoken to a number of past students and they all say the same thing. "I loved going to C3 because you were always there and would amuse me." In the time-out room we had to write in a book what we had done wrong. These past students also said they loved it even more when they read the C3 Book. It was a detailed record of all the things I had done, a record of all the less memorable achievements in life.

During Year Seven I faced my first challenge in taking medication. Every morning my mother made my breakfast. Neatly laid out was food, Ritalin, asthma tablets and two types of asthma inhalers. This was my daily routine and still is today. It does not worry me that I have to do this every day. It has been a part of my life since I was eight. The way I see it, I need to take asthma medication every day so I don't die, so there is no difference in taking Ritalin to stop people wanting me to die! That's a joke!

The problem was my lunch time dosage—I didn't take it! This was a big problem during school and even in Year Twelve. My mother put the Ritalin in a small film canister with my lunch, because I was embarrassed, and if anyone asked what the tablet was for, I would say it was for asthma. At school I developed such a sneaky technique of taking my Ritalin at lunch time that people never asked or even saw me take it when I was taking it right in front of them. My friends always used to take my drink from my school bag and it used to annoy me, because I had no liquid to swallow my tablets. It is pretty hard taking tablets with water from a water fountain. In theory, this should have worked, but it didn't. After being confined in a classroom for a couple of hours I was like a caged bull. When the bell went I burst out of the classroom and hit the oval to burn off energy. It was time to run, play and sometimes fight.

Claims that Ritalin suppresses the appetite are pretty much true in my case. I rarely worried about lunch at school because of the side effects of Ritalin. That's not 100 per cent correct. When I take Ritalin I lose my appetite for normal food, such as the lunch my mother made for me. I would often buy more exciting things from the cafeteria and in doing so forget to or not bother to take my medication. This side effect of Ritalin is somewhat strange. I feel hungry because I am weak and have hunger pains but I won't eat. I eat a little, but I find myself picking at my food and often either throw it or give it away. The consequences of missing my lunchtime medication usually resulted in my behavior becoming erratic and uncontrollable in afternoon classes.

I don't like being different!

While at the school I encountered my first experience of everyone knowing what was wrong with me. A girl had an eating disorder—well, I thought she had an eating disorder. I'm not quite sure but at the time if I thought something, then to me it was true. I would tease her about this and told everyone. I thought she was just doing it for attention. The student counselor advised the girl to say, when I next said something to her, 'Well, I know what is wrong with you!' I was so angry I came home and went ballistic at my mother. I told her I didn't want the school to know because this was exactly what I had thought would happen—my embarrassing secret was out. However, I was wrong. The school had not told the girl what was wrong with me. My parents, the school counselor, the girl involved and I had a meeting. Before then she didn't know that I had ADD but now she did and from then on the whole school knew. From that day forward, both teachers and students treated me differently. Instead of me being the one picking on other kids, they now had a powerful weapon to use against me, and they did. If I teased anyone

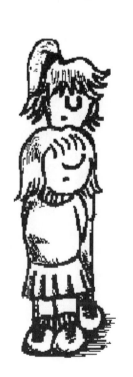
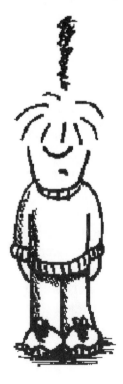

they would throw it back in my face. Parents must take this possibility into account when they tell people that their son has ADD.

The child already feels different and has low self-esteem. If his peer group yells, "He's got ADD!" his self-esteem and self-perception are further lowered. But if you don't tell the school, how will the school and teachers understand your child's behavior and specific needs? I suggest telling schools after you have stressed that only the teachers are to know. Do not tell the parents of your son's peer group. People talk and people can be very nasty. You must remember that your son does not want to be different but realizes he is. By telling everyone, you just create a bigger problem for him.

Teachers are not trained in dealing with students who have ADD. They often try ludicrous strategies that do not work and force the student to persist with them. For example, once a teacher gave me an elastic band and every time I did something impulsive I was to flick the elastic band around my wrist to remind me to control myself. I tried this but it did nothing for my impulsivity, it was just another tool to amuse myself with in class. Every time I was bored or lacked concentration, I would flick the student next to me or shoot it across the room and hit someone. But the teachers could not take the elastic band off me because it was meant to help me! Another advantage was in having an unlimited supply of elastic bands to fire at people on the bus, out of the bus, walking to the train station, people on the train, and when I was home I had my family and pets to fire at. You would think that this strategy would have ceased because of its ineffectiveness. But no, I had to persist with this strategy, ridiculous as it was. If something does not work with your child, try something else. It is for reasons such as this I decided to undertake the challenge of writing this book.

Letters to parents and semester one report card!

Dear Mr. and Mrs. Polis,

I am writing to inform you about some behavior of Ben's that I felt you would want to know about. It was brought to my attention that Ben has been telling jokes to other students, the nature of which could be only termed as offensive.

Recently I held a discussion with Ben and some other students about using language that would fit into the category of sexist terminology. While Ben was not the only one involved it was very clearly impressed upon him that such behavior is totally unacceptable.

Given the nature of the "jokes" Ben has been telling and that some were directed towards female students it would appear he has disregarded my warning. Ben has been constantly advised about more appropriate ways to behave towards fellow students but he does experience difficulty in following such advice. In order to better monitor Ben's behavior I will be placing him on a conduct card. Staff will be asked to write a descriptive comment on his card for each lesson. Ben should present this card at home each night for you to read and sign.

As a consequence for his telling of jokes of an unacceptable nature, I will restrict Ben to one area of the school for one week. My aim in doing this is to make the point to him that if he cannot control his behavior in an appropriate manner, he will be observed. Hopefully, he will come to see that in order to move freely around the school he must adopt a more responsible approach.

Could I ask that you telephone me at the school so that we can discuss this matter further? My apologies for sending such a long, handwritten letter but I did want this to reach home today.

Thank you for your support in this matter,

Year Seven Co-ordinator

9th December 1994

Dear Mr. and Mrs. Polis,

Unfortunately on Friday 9th December, Ben was involved in a fighting incident at school. The consequence of this action is that Ben will be suspended out of school from Monday 12th December, to Wednesday 14th December (three days).

The school has a policy of no fighting and as this is Ben's second offense, he has been suspended for three days.

If you have any queries regarding this matter don't hesitate to contact me at school.

Yours Faithfully

YEAR SEVEN CO-ORDINATOR

GENERAL COMMENTS FROM REPORT CARD:

Music: Ben is continually calling out, attention seeking and disrupting the class.

French: Ben has not focused on his work even when redirected to it. His assignment is mostly up to date, but other work has been neglected.

English: Ben has indicated that he does have some ability in his area. Inconsistency works against Ben and until he adopts strategies and listens to advice offered aimed at helping him, he will not gain the best possible outcomes.

The term one report card is all I have from Year Seven. I was meant to get my final report card, however it was not to be. Let me tell you why. By the end of Year Seven I had had enough of the secondary college and they had had enough of me. School had finished for the year and I had not yet picked up my report card. My mother and I were going shopping and on our way there we decided to pick up my report card and books from my locker. At the front office I asked to see the Year Seven coordinator. She said, "Who do you think you are, arriving at school without an appointment, out of uniform etc?" I told her the school year was finished, therefore I did not have to wear a uniform now, I just wanted my report and would then leave. She told me I would have to wait until three o'clock, about two hours. I replied that I wanted it now because my mother was waiting. She said my mother would have to wait and I would have to sit in the office for the two hours and wait. I was not going to play her game so I told her that she could keep my report card and walked off to get my books from the locker. She stood there and yelled at the top of her lungs, "Benjamin Polis! Come back here! You are not going anywhere!" She followed me to my locker and again demanded that I refrain from leaving. I did not say a word. She had no control over me, she knew it. I exploited it and loved being in control of the situation. I didn't care. I was going to another school the following year and her threats did not matter. With my books, I walked out of that school with her still following me, still yelling, jumped into my mother's car and drove off. I did not care then and still don't care now. I was glad to be out of the school and have not been back since. As I said in the start of this chapter, Year Seven was probably the worst year of my life, academically, mentally, socially, with self-esteem, and not to mention behaviorally.

Camp chaos!

During the summer holidays my mother sought peace and quiet by sending me to a Christian camp. It was an opportunity for underprivileged children whose parents could not afford a holiday for them, along with many others just there to have a good time. After the disaster of my first year in secondary school I was mentally unstable and very angry.

On the second day I lost total control. I was quietly sitting on my bunk when another boy started hitting me with a broomstick, just to get a reaction. He got one, all right! With extreme force I grabbed the broomstick off him and repeatedly smashed it over

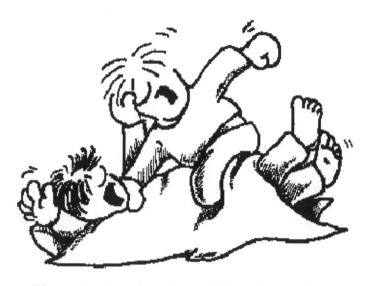

him, yelling at the top of my lungs, "How do you like it, PUNK?" The leader, who was much older and stronger, finally restrained me. My impulsive behavior and temper were out of control.

The following day a girl started teasing me about bashing someone with a broomstick. I told her, "F*@# off! You're just a stupid fat cow!" She hit me in the face. I lost it again. With one all-mighty swing I knocked her out! I'm not proud of this, especially because she was a girl. However, an angry and impulsive boy with ADD does not think about what he is doing and doesn't understand why he is acting in such a manner. I do know why I was so mentally unstable during this part of my life. I hated myself and I hated everyone else. My parents had sent me away like some kind of condemned criminal. I didn't want to go to the stupid camp and I hated everyone there. But most of all I hated myself. I was about to go to my fifth school at the age of thirteen. I felt as though no one liked me and now even my family couldn't handle me any more. Along with this, I was in a very unfamiliar environment. My ordered routine was not there and I didn't have my mother to do everything for me. Camps and I don't really work well. As a matter of fact, every school camp I have been on, my mother would have to drive back and pick me up! She liked the thought of me going away but she hated it because she always knew that she would have to drive out in about three days to pick me up.

The funny thing is that on this camp I met one of my best friends. His name was Jared Smith. He was really sick on this camp and lay in bed for about five days. He was obviously bored and wanted some stimulation. As he got better he thought he would have a go at setting me up as well. Not a good idea! I don't remember exactly what happened but I do remember what I did. I jumped on top of him as he lay in bed and punched him up! So if you look at my stats, the camp went for five days and I knocked out three people in five days! Not bad! In the following chapter I will tell you how Jared and I became friends.

Another example of a camp not going down too well was my Year Seven camp. This camp was absolutely wild. The teachers' camp was about five hundred meters away from the students. The students were meant to sleep in these old trains converted into dorms. However, no one slept! If you can imagine about a hundred and fifty kids running wild at about three in the morning jumping on top of the trains and just being foolish, that was camp. However, it was during this camp I had my first experience with a girl. It is pretty funny looking back on it now. See, I was set up with this girl, like you are in Year Seven and we had to kiss. I had never really kissed a girl before and didn't have a clue. Well anyway, we started to kiss and she didn't stop! The problem was it was cold outside and I had a bit of asthma. I breathe through my mouth like a lot of asthmatics and when this girl was kissing me I couldn't breathe. I pulled away and started to cough. I think I am the only person in the world to have an asthma attack from kissing.

But this is not why I got into trouble. The girl and I slept in the same bed that night, but nothing happened sexually. Anyway, the following morning she told the Year Seven coordinator, "I slept with Ben Polis last night." Well, she took it totally out of context. We were sent home that day and my mother once again had to come and pick me up. We were both made examples of and sent home because the teachers were so angry because all the students had been out partying the night before. I didn't really mind being sent home anyway, the camp was crap! When my mother came to pick me up she was so angry. She wouldn't even buy me McDonald's on the way home when she bought my sister McDonald's. I was in soooooooooo much trouble again!

Catholic college

The choice of this college by my mother was an excellent one. The criteria she used to choose my new school were simple but quite brilliant. The school had to be small enough so that I got the necessary attention that was lacking at larger schools. An all-boys' school was also very important to limit distractions from my crutch area. She found my new school and I am eternally grateful that she found this college. Let me tell you a little bit about this great school.

I believe this is the best school I have been to out of a possible five other candidates. The reason is very simple. It is a small Catholic school of around four hundred boys. It only goes from Year Seven to 10, which allows a lot of personal attention for students both capable and not so capable. I believe the big difference between this school and other schools is that the teachers just simply care a lot more about their students. Discipline is enforced and you really can't get away with a lot because everyone

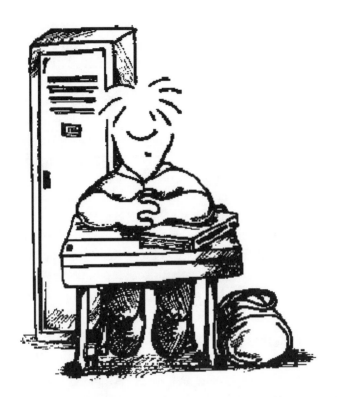

knows everyone. It did not matter if you were a Year Seven kid, it was quite acceptable to hang out with students in Year Ten. I had never been to a school such as this. The school also had a very diverse cultural base of students. Again, it did not matter where you were from. Prejudices did not arise.

On a personal note, this school was perfect for me. Unlike other schools where you had to move from class to class, the teachers came to you. Some students may not like this idea but I think it is fantastic. You had the same desk and sat next to the same person every day. You had your own personal space, which was yours for the whole year. These were not permanently set out but it was an unwritten class rule. This is especially great for an ADD child because your own personal space allows you to settle in at the start of the day. This allows you to get off to a great start. At the previous college, if I forgot a book I would have to put my hand up and ask to get it from my locker. This would annoy the teachers and then I would have to run to my locker so I wouldn't fall behind in the period. However, there, if I forgot a book all I would have to do was walk two meters behind me and go to my locker. That's what I call efficiency. I feel its greatest attribute is not that it is a small school or even its great academic record but that it gives kids a second and third chance and persists with troubled students. The school had many students who had been expelled from other schools. Unlike other schools that shifted the problem on, they took the time to resolve the problem. If there were more schools like that in Australia the level of academic achievement would increase dramatically.

Year Eight at the college

For the first time in my school life I decided to adopt a new radical concept. I was going to try! At first I hated going there. However, I liked it better than the previous college. No one knew me and I could start off fresh—and I did. I tried hard, I behaved and I did homework for the first time in my life. However this smoke screen would soon be unmasked. His name was Jared Smith and he blew my cover! He was the same boy I had bashed at Christian camp only a couple of months earlier. I did not remember him or even remember bashing him up, until he confronted me one day at school. I didn't have any friends at the time and remember talking to a Down's Syndrome student named Paul on my first day. Jared was also a new student in Year Eight and was in the same position I was in. However, he had made friends a lot easier than me at first.

The reason I had not made any friends was not lack of social skills. It was due to the new Ben, the quiet and settled Ben. I lay low for the first couple of weeks and did not intrude on anyone. This was the reason I had not made any friends—until Jared opened his big mouth!

When he confronted me a couple of weeks into the first term I remember exactly what he said. "Are you Ben Polis from—?" "No, of course not!" I replied with a cheeky grin! My cover was blown big time! We became good friends from that day forward. A couple of weeks later he told me that he had seen me on the first day and crapped himself and walked the other way. He told me that he couldn't believe his eyes, thinking to himself, "A new school and I am stuck with a psycho!" I had not realized that he had already been telling people that I was a little crazy and that I had beaten up half of the camp! I guess this is the reason that no one wanted to be my friend. After a while people realized that I wasn't crazy and they all wanted to talk to me. I guess they were intrigued after the stories Jared had told them. After that I made heaps of friends.

It was during Year Eight that I uncovered a gift that I hadn't really used. I had always been a great athlete in primary school but didn't really think much of it because I was competing against a handful of students. Well, the annual athletics day was coming up and I was pretty cocky that I would win! Like all things, I guess, in life, I just have this self-perception that I am the best even if I am not. This allows me to believe in myself and at the same time improves my self-esteem. I had already sorted out my competition, and his name was Tim Prescott, the fastest kid in Year Eight. I had challenged him verbally in school that I was going to kill him on the running track. This went down very well. A bit of rivalry from the new kid to knock off the reigning champion was just the ticket I needed to make a name for myself. Well, the big day came and Melbourne turned on the weather the only way Melbourne can. It rained and it was washed out. The school rescheduled it again and the Melbourne weather turned it on again. It rained harder than last time. The showdown the school was waiting for was not going to happen.

The school athletics day is the qualifying one for the interschool athletics day. The problem was that I could not qualify. So Tim was chosen for all the events on the previous year's performance. I threw up a stink over this and I was allowed to run the two hundred meters in the interschool athletics championships. This was not well perceived by the other students. Who does this new kid think he is, telling his new school that he is running in the two hundred meters? I didn't care—I put on an image of invincibility.

The big day came. I borrowed Jared's spikes, which were about two sizes too small. People would not have known it but I was scared. I had convinced this new school that I was the best thing since sliced bread. But I didn't even know if I could win! Well, the

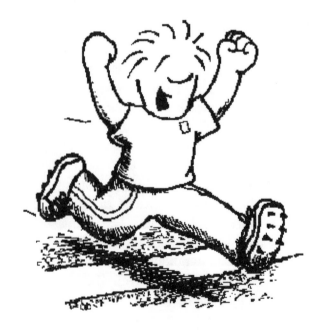

big day was here, and it was make or break time. I was either going to be a hero or be labeled as a loser like I had been at secondary college. I was determined to win at any cost!

I lined up on the blocks with the whole school watching me. Because it was such a small school all the students and teachers were allowed to come and cheer us on. The starter's gun fired! Bang! F*@#! I had false started! I guess that was my impulsiveness again shining through. I lined up again but this time I started perfectly. I ran like I had never run before! I remember going into the eighty-meter bend coming about third! When I got around the last bend, and with about another eight metres to go, I was in front by about two meters. The crowd was going wild! Spurred on by this, I increased my lead even more. I couldn't see any of the other runners—I had left them for dead. I finished in first place with my arms up in the air like Michael Johnson at the Atlanta Olympic Games. I won by a huge margin—about seven meters! I had done it! I had believed I could and I did! I had to do it!

After I finished I was approached by one of the marshals. At the time I was talking to the school principal. The marshal asked me, "Do you run?" "Yes, but only from my mum!" I then replied, "No, I have never run before for a club." "Well, you should, you nearly broke the interschool record." She took down my phone number and my running career was started. I ran straight to a public phone box to call my mum. I told her what I had achieved. She was so pleased! I'm not sure if she was most pleased at me winning or that in her son's whole schooling life he was finally happy!

After I had finished talking to my mother I went and sat with the other students. I was suddenly being approached by teachers, parents and students, all congratulating me on my performance. I then asked—no that's not true, I demanded—that I choose other events that I wanted to do. I then went on to win the 100m, 400m, high jump, javelin and the 4x100m relay. Our Year Eight athletic team won the championship for their year level. Thanks to me! The following day I went to school and people kept congratulating me! I loved it! The only downside was I had created a nickname for myself that I was not too fond of—Roids! There was a rumor going around the school that I was on steroids! How pathetic, would you believe that a fourteen-year-old boy would be doing steroids? Hello, this is not East Germany!

I sailed through Year Eight with average marks. No real trouble or anything too alarming. For the first time in my whole life I had found a school that accepted me and I started to love going to school. My behavior at home improved greatly and my bursts of anger were not so prevalent. It's strange when you think about it. Parents are always asking questions. Why is their son acting in such an abnormal manner? However, from my personal experience, I believe as a parent you must look at your son's environment. If he has low self-esteem because he can't read like the other students, gets into trouble and can't make friends because he is not accepted because of his erratic behavior, you must resolve these issues first if you want to improve your son's behavior. I have a belief that people who fight and are angry do so because they are unhappy with their own perception of themselves. When I was younger I was getting into fights in and out of school. But when I was happy with my own self-perception these ADHD symptoms were not as dominant—just something to think about in your own child's environment.

My report card from Year Eight showed some great improvements in my academic and behavioral performance— especially when you look at my performance in Year Seven when I didn't pass a subject. Year Eight was a real learning experience for me. It was during this age that I started to learn the foundations of my many self-help techniques, which I will discuss in the later chapters. Another important fact that I learned in Year Eight was that self-esteem and just basically feeling good about yourself really contribute to overall improvements in behavior. This is even more important in an ADD child. An unhappy ADD child will always make everyone else around him unhappy. So again I am reinforcing that it is fundamentally important to look at your child's social environment.

Bad boy Ben is back!

Year Nine was without a doubt my worst year. It really doesn't make sense since I had had such a fantastic year in Year Eight. My grades had improved; I even passed all my subjects for the first time in my life. My behavior was nearly perfect, well, as perfect as an ADHD child's behavior can be. Well, you might be wondering, what the hell happened in a couple of months? You'd better hang on to your seats because my life is about to get ugly!

Year Nine started like every other year. Your year level has an assembly where your coordinators lecture you for hours about the same thing every year. "This is one of the most important years of your schooling life and you must make a more concentrated effort with your studies! Blah, blah blah!" Well, unlike the year before, I had made a concentrated decision not to take my studies seriously ,or life in general. This is not something that I recommend to anyone! Because the only thing I successfully achieved in Year Nine was to successfully *f*@# up* my life!

Again, like in Year Seven, I was out of control. However, there was a big difference between Year Seven and Year Nine. The big difference was that in Year Seven I did not know any better. I was always like that and I had come to the conclusion that I was out of control and I could not change that. But this time I was out of

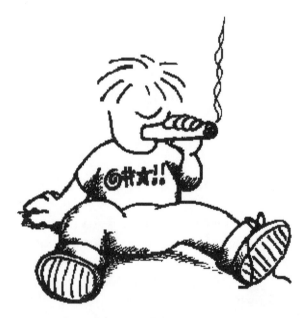

control because I had deliberately chosen to be. I knew I could behave and be an asset to my school and society. I had done it and I had done it all by myself without anyone else's help. I had no secret pill that changed me into a perfect student. The only secret that I had uncovered was self-control. I had chosen to take control over my behavior and subsequently my life. I like to refer to this as, "I was in control of my brain instead of my brain controlling me!" However, in Year Nine I chose to let my brain once again control me!

This thought process and change in my behavior I believe to be the result of a number of factors. I had become a parent's worst nightmare. I was a fifteen-year-old, rebellious, know-it-all teenager. I was rebelling against everyone and everything. Authority was my arch-enemy and I was determined to crush it! However, this was not to be. Authority won with a quick and decisive battle. So if I can paint a picture of myself at the time I had very dangerous personality traits.

I was:

Impulsive
Angry
Smarty pants
Conceited
Extremely violent
Very intelligent
Manipulative
Horny teenager controlled by my crutch!
Rebellious

As you can see, I was again my worst enemy. It was not my ADHD, it was my way of thinking. My ADHD only highlighted my very dangerous personality traits. I lasted only about five weeks into the term before I was suspended. I was in a fighting incident with an older boy in Year Ten. I gave him a beating, though. I guess looking back on it now I was not fighting him because I didn't like him. I had a point to prove. I wanted to be *Bad Boy Ben*! This extremely aggressive and self-destroying attitude of mine followed everywhere I went. I would get into fights at school, coming home from school, on the weekends and at home. My answer to all my problems was to do what I do best—be impulsive, which meant fighting in a lot of cases.

The school by this time had had enough of me. I was put on probation at school and got a daily report card. This report card is a good idea. It is also an excellent idea for parents with children who have ADD. How it works is quite simple. Every class your son gets this report card signed with comments from that teacher. Then he brings it home for you to sign. It gives a running commentary on your son's daily life.

When thinking about Year Nine I always tell people of my love-hate relationship with my math teacher. He hated me and I loved him hating me! He had a very distinctive voice, which I could mimic perfectly. Every time he would yell at me I would reply in his voice. "Yes, Mr —!" It made him go wild and my fellow students loved it because it was so funny. But the funny thing about this relationship between him and I was that we had an unspoken language. I knew what he was thinking and he knew what I was thinking. My math class was such a repetitive experience, it always went like this. I had one warning before I was kicked out of the class. But I was not told verbally that I had been given a warning, it was just a look and I knew that look. But when I did something else disruptive the second time there was no yelling or anything said. I knew it and he knew it. He would then walk over to my desk as cool as a cucumber and get one side of the table and I would get the other side and we would carry my table outside together. But remember, this was all done with nothing said to each other. The students would laugh because it worked like clockwork and it happened every lesson.

It was during Year Nine that I started to experiment with alcohol and marijuana. Now this is a tip for all parents out there. All kids experiment with booze and drugs! If you decide to turn a blind eye to this problem you are only encouraging it! If you think it's hard for your child to get booze it's not! But the surprising thing is that kids can often get drugs more easily than booze. You don't have to be eighteen or twenty-one to buy drugs. There is no age limit for buying drugs. The only thing you need is money! Well, I started to experiment with marijuana. I even attempted to grow some. At the time, my mother would tease me because they would always die. She told me about two years later that they had died because she was spraying them with weed killer. Anyway, that's not my point. This is my point! If you look at the personality traits I had at the time and then add a combination of drugs and alcohol you have yourself a recipe for disaster.

I remember one night very clearly. It was a Friday night and a couple of friends and I were smoking pot in my bedroom. My mother came in and could smell it. She went ballistic, screaming and yelling at me. She told the other boys that she was going to ring their mothers. This triggered something off in my head and I went absolutely crazy! I kicked the front door in and swore the most vulgar of profanities at my mother. I walked out the front gate with my father in hot pursuit. I turned around and picked up an extremely heavy flower pot and threw it at my father. He moved in the nick of time and it exploded on impact. My friends and I walked to the closest train station. My father had jumped into his car and was following me. He caught up with me about fifty meters from the train station. He pulled over next to me and told me to get into the car. I ran up and started to punch my father in the head through the driver's side window. I kicked the driver's side door in. I then ran off with my friends as if nothing had happened. The following day my father tried to get a restraining order on me. My mother would not let him go through with it. I don't understand how it would have worked anyway, because we both live under the same roof.

I am certainly not proud of this incident and it seems unbelievable when I think about it today. However, it happened and I did do it. I could leave things out of this book that I am embarrassed about, such as this, but they happened and I did them. It was a part of my life and I don't believe that the truth should be manipulated to cover my embarrassment. I have thought about this incident a number of times since. I do not put it down to having ADHD. I have no proof of this statement that I am about to make but I believe it to be true. For some reason unknown to me, when I use marijuana it changes the chemicals in my brain. I have discussed this with other ADHD people and they also believe this to be true. Marijuana, I believe, should not be the drug of choice for an ADHD person. It makes you go crazy without you even realizing it. I am not against marijuana and believe it should be legalized for medical purposes. However, I strongly recommend that if you have ADHD or your child does you should stay clear of it.

During Year Nine I constantly challenged my boundaries at college. I was on probation and I decided that I would not change my ways. I continued causing trouble at school and fighting. The school had had enough this time. I was playing Australian Rules Football at lunch time. It was a favorite pastime there. Quite often we played with fifty plus kids from all year levels. It was quite funny, though. Because of the cultural diversity most of the boys did not have a clue how to play. We had Vietnamese boys, Greek, Italian, Yugoslavs, Cambodians, etc. So we played a game that resembled more of a Roman battle at the Coliseum. Rough and tough were basically the only rules. When someone was tackled and brought to the ground the call would go out! "Stakes On!" You would have anywhere from ten to thirty boys jumping on someone. It was great!

Anyway, this day I was dominating the game as usual, kicking goals and playing as roughly as I could. I was playing on a new boy to the school who had a bit of a name as a good footballer. I didn't think much of him and was out-marking him at every opportunity. He didn't like this and I was stirring him up. Anyway, it all got a bit heated, as it did during these games on the oval. Well, he and I had been shaping up to each other for months. We had a small fight, nothing over the top. But the only thing the teacher on duty saw was me swing at him. I was suspended once again but this time it was very different. The school called my father and I up to the school at the end of the day. I was told that I had to find a new school. I burst into tears, I couldn't believe it—they were serious this time. I loved it there, it was the best school I had ever been to and I had never thought they would expel me! I was told to try and find a new school and if I couldn't I was to ring them. The school insisted that *I* was to find a new school, not my parents. I did try to find a new school but no-one wanted me—funny about that! Anyway, I had already been to all the schools in my area and my college was about forty minutes' train ride away already. Mum jokes about it today, saying things like, "I thought you would end up going to school on the other side of Melbourne!"

The college is very dear to my heart and I was not going to let them throw me out. I had a real change of heart during this time in my life. I had finally realized that I had been biting the hand that fed me. I wrote this letter to the school pleading to be reinstated as a student:

> — College,
>
> To Mr. —,
>
> I have thought about my actions leading up to my suspension (being asked to leave). I have come to the conclusion that I have not been acting in an appropriate way to my teachers. I know now that I should have treated them with more respect and listened to what they have been saying over the past couple of months. I would like to come back and try to become a better student than I have been in the past.
>
> Yours sincerely,
>
> Benjamin Polis

Here is the letter the college sent me in reply.

> 17th September, 1996
>
> Dear Mr. and Mrs. Polis
>
> Following our conversation, the College is prepared to allow Ben to continue his education here next semester under the following conditions:
>
> It is required that Ben give an undertaking not to be involved or associated with any form of intimidation,

bullying, verbal or physical harassment of any member of this College community, student or staff. As a member of the College community, his conduct with the general public must be appropriate.

Ben will be on probation for the remainder of this year. It is our present intention that in the middle of next term, a meeting will take place, at which his academic progress and conduct will be discussed. If satisfactory progress has been made, Ben's position will be reviewed.

Any involvement in the activities mentioned above, which come to the College's attention, will result in Ben's position being reviewed, and you may be asked to withdraw Ben from the College.

This letter is to be signed by you, the parents, Ben himself and returned at the start of next term.

Yours sincerely,

—

Principal

As you can see, the college did give me a second chance once again. I could not find another school that would accept me. The strict rules above on my reinstatement were very hard to keep, as I found in the following year. I was not allowed to come back at that time but I would be allowed to come back the next year, in Year Ten. During Year Nine I was suspended for over two months all up, on about eight different occasions. I would again like to thank the college for giving me a second chance after many previous chances. Likewise I would like to highlight the tremendous support the college offers to students like me. It provides a vital service to the overall improvement of the social and educational development of the youth of Victoria. Australia would be a lot better off if there were more schools that displayed this caring approach to their students.

My report from Year Nine was not very good, as you can imagine. I will not bore you with the details. However it went a little bit like this.

English
Due to Ben's many absences, it is difficult to accurately assess him in this subject. When work is submitted it is of a very good standard, and reflects considerable thought, but it is often late and therefore marked as such. He needs to improve his organizational skills and submit work on time.
A disappointing effort!'

Looking back on my report from Year Nine made me realize something that I had not really understood until I was much older. All my grades for class work in my report were extremely poor, often Es and Ds. However, my test grades were in the high nineties. It seems a bit strange, but not for an ADHD student. The problem is quite simple. In class I cannot concentrate or stay on task due to the working environment. But when I do an exam I can concentrate because of the settled working environment. Along with this, you have to concentrate when doing an exam. So does this mean that I have selective concentration difficulties. Do I think so? No, I know so! Just something to think about with your child's own education. Maybe you should look at his working environment in closer detail. You may see a huge improvement as I did in Year Twelve, which I will discuss in greater detail.

At this age I was also accused of burning down a local football club. I remember the day very clearly. It was seven o'clock in the morning and Mum woke me up to tell me the CIB, the detective police, were at the front door. Six detectives in black trench coats confronted me. Someone had told them that I had burned down the local football club. This is just another example of my bad reputation in the area. I did not do it but the police were sure it was me. I eventually proved my innocence because I was at work when it happened. But I learned something from all this. I can now see why people who are innocent of a crime admit to it. When all this was happening, for a little while, the police convinced me that I had done it. But I just stuck to my guns and told them if that they thought I had done it, it was their job to prove it! They never did and I thank God that he made me a strong enough person to not give in to the massive pressure I was under.

Year Ten!

During Year Ten nothing really changed much. I was still Ben Polis and I was still acting like the class clown. I was not as bad as I was in Year Nine but there was not much difference. However, there was one very important difference. This time I was on probation. Any false move and I was out. This threat constantly lingering over my head all the time did deter me somewhat. It was during Year Ten that I found out that I had some very strong allies. The first was my Year Nine English and drama teacher. She had constantly put her neck out in my defense in Year Nine. But I did not have her in Year Ten to mother me, as she had in Year Nine. Still, in Year Ten I was not alone. My home room teacher was the best teacher I have ever had! I found out in Year Ten that the school had wanted me to leave but he had volunteered his very brave services to be my homeroom teacher and English teacher. Without the support of these two teachers I feel my life would have not turned out the way it is today. Thank you!

Here is a letter he sent when I told him I was writing this book.

When you enter the teaching profession, nobody warns you about the multitude of personalities that you will confront, day in day out. It's strange how over the years, you remember certain students. The bright one, the funny one, the rude one, the challenging one, and the poetic one ... Ben Polis was all of these.

I was only in my second year of teaching, when I learned that Ben was going to be in my class. An involuntary shudder passed through my body. Ben was the loud one in the yard. Restless, energetic, ringleader, exhausting, confronting. In short, Ben was hard work.

Sometimes when you teach, you have to get beyond (or beneath? or through?) the disruptive behavior and get to know the individual. Although there were times when Ben could be maddening—what 15-year-old isn't?—I got to know him. It was worth the effort. Ben could give the impression that he was uninterested, disorganized and a disaster waiting to happen. In truth, there thrived a keen intellect, an ability to think clearly and an articulate young man.

So how did I cope with Ben?

A lot of it was trial and error. I tried a variety of teaching strategies and approaches, sometimes in consultation with Ben. I certainly learned a lot through having Ben in my classes.

In order to keep Ben engaged, tasks had to be short, sharp and hands on. For instance, when teaching essay structures, Ben didn't cope with the simple chalk and talk approach. He showed real progress, however, when he could cut an essay up into its constituent parts, label them and use them as a model for his own writing.

In a similar way, Ben responded to visual and aural stimuli. He could, for instance, listen to a piece of music or look at a photo and then write a short piece. The key, it seemed to me, was to break up the lessons, so that he could avoid being bored. The other key was to set clearly defined parameters for him: "We'll listen to a piece of music, then I'd like you to write two stanzas." This worked well for Ben.

It was equally important that Ben learned to work within the guidelines that the rest of the class worked within, hands up, etc. Keeping Ben on task was a battle. At times, he would lose the plot. Perhaps the thing that was most effective, at these times, was giving him choices. "Ben, if you continue to talk and to interrupt the class, I will have to move you to the front ...", "to write in your diary ..." "to ask you to leave the room ..." etc. This allowed Ben to take responsibility for his own actions and the consequences of those actions. The fact that I had built a relationship with him gave me some referential power over him. I tried to ensure that I would criticize his behavior rather than to express my disappointment in him. For the most part, this worked well.

When Ben graduated, I was genuinely proud of him. He had worked hard under trying circumstances. There were times when I really wondered if he'd ever make it. It's so wonderful to see the great adult that he has become.

May 30, 2001

In Year Ten my academic performances did improve. I had chosen to do a Year Eleven subject in Year Ten. The subject was Year Eleven mathematics, which is quite funny because I failed Year Nine maths with flying colors. This was the vice-principal's idea to encourage me and relieve some of the boredom I was constantly complaining about at school. It worked quite well. When I am challenged I concentrate and stay on task better. If something is easy I amuse myself in class, often annoying the teacher with disruptive behavior. This is something to think about with your child. If you expect an ADHD child to sit still with no mental or physical challenge you have no chance. So you should always have a bag of toys or books and so on to stimulate your child. This will make your life a bit easier.

My academic standing did improve but my behavior did not improve drastically. I was still getting in trouble, but I was not failing as I had in Year Nine. My work was often handed in late because I was so unorganized, but I got it in. This was a problem of mine throughout my whole school life, including Year Twelve. Below are some letters to my parents from the college.

> Dear Mr. and Mrs. Polis,
>
> I am writing to you to let you know that Ben made a very unpleasant comment to me today in my classroom. Ben is no longer actually in my class, he simply walked into it—P6—today.
>
> I am quite a tolerant person with a reasonable sense of humor. I am not averse to a little friendly banter but I am not used to foul remarks, masked as jokes, being directed at me.
>
> I was offended and disgusted. I require a written apology from him at least. I will contact you further, next week.

This letter does not tell the real story. See, I had been kicked out of class because of disruptive behavior, most probably because I was bored in class. The problem with this disciplinary technique is I was sent outside to an even more mind-numbing environment. So like any ADHD child I amused myself. I started to approach the classrooms in the corridor, where I was meant to be sitting. I was pretending to be a door-to-door salesmen. I was selling exercise bikes going cheap. The catch was that I approached all the larger teachers who I had identified as my target market. But the reason the exercise bikes were so cheap was that they were

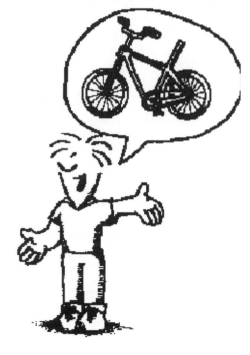

missing a seat, which I used as a selling point. The seat-less exercise bikes offered sexual stimulation to keep you exercising. The students were in hysterics and the teachers were after my head. That's the real story. But it's funny how teachers always have such a pleasant way of retelling stories when it gets to your parents.

Dear Mr. and Mrs. Polis,

Due to poor behavior at the canteen over the last few weeks and the showing of disrespect for its manageress, Ben is not allowed to enter the canteen for all of next week. He will not be allowed to enter the canteen following that until he has passed on to me a letter of apology for her.

Year level coordinator.

The funny thing about this whole situation was that I got my friends to buy my lunch from the canteen and then subsequently stuffed myself in front of the canteen lady to annoy her. Also, I never wrote that apology, but I probably should have. So here goes.

Dear Mrs. —

I am sorry for my disrespectful behavior directed at you in 1997.

19th May 1997

Dear Mr. and Mrs. Polis,

As I indicated in our telephone conversation earlier today, and after consultation with the Principal and the Year Ten coordinator, Ben has been suspended from the College for an incident which took place on Ventura Bus No. 703 on the morning of Monday 19th May.

The incident concerned an exchange between Ben and a group of disabled persons who regularly use this bus. A parent of a student who will be attending the College in 1998 was most upset and telephoned the College to convey his dismay at Ben's behavior. It is of concern to us that the image of the College has been tarnished and Ben's insensitivity to the needs of disabled persons has been highlighted.

Both the principal and myself hope that Ben realizes that as he is making decisions for next year, incidents such as today's may have an impact on the College's willingness to recommend that Ben continue his education elsewhere in 1998.

Yours sincerely,

Deputy principal

At the bottom of this letter I found a note attached to it by my father. It states that I was suspended again just before the end of the school year and had to pick up my report after all the other students had left. So I could not incite students into more rebellious behavior.

Well, it was true that I had insulted these disabled passengers on the school bus. However, they were asking for it. These two disabled people were a couple. But they were not quiet little disabled people as the school had thought. They were loud-mouthed, rude fruit loops. They had names for every bus they went on and thought they owned the bus, literally. The reason I had insulted this couple was they were insulting the students of the college, saying they were a bunch of dills, and so on. So as you can see they were not totally innocent. However, I should have bitten my tongue and stayed out of this, which would have gone against all of my ADHD impulses. But the funny thing that did come to mind out of reading this letter was that it reminded me of something else.

Every time I would get on a bus throughout my school life every bus driver knew my name. They would say things like, "Ben, are we going to have a good day today?" I thought this was pretty funny because I had never told them my name but they knew who I was. Along with this, about a year ago this lady on the train said, "Hi Ben, how you been?" I looked at her and said, "Who the hell are you?" She said I didn't know her but she knew me. The lady had caught the same train as me for three years. She told me that she would recite my daily routine, of calling out on the train and so on, to her friends at work during morning tea. She also told me that I had developed a cult following in her office and they were bitterly disappointed when I was not on the train. I guess I made their day go a bit faster. So I guess we do need people like me because the world would be a very boring place without ADHD people.

25th August, 1997
Mr. and Mrs. Polis,
I am writing to express my growing concern regarding Ben's attitude and behavior in class.

After discussions between your son's teachers, and his homeroom teacher, it has become necessary to again inform you of our concerns, particularly Ben's disruptive, antagonistic, intimidating and at times aggressive behavior in class.

It is of concern to us that Ben's behavior is reflected in his poor attitude to his school work and of greater concern is the effect that your son's behavior is having on other members of his class. Every member of the community has the right to learn. At present Ben is not respecting the right of other students to learn.

The decision has been taken that if Ben's behavior continues to have a detrimental effect on the learning environment of the College and other students or is in any way intimidating to either staff or students, he will be withdrawn from classes and have no further contact with the student body. This suspension from classes will be for a period of one or more days. During this time Ben will be given all work by the class teacher and will be expected to complete the work.

After the period of withdrawal from classes has been served, and after discussion between you and yourselves Ben will be allowed to resume classes. If Ben's behavior continues to be disruptive Ben may be suspended from the College. In this circumstance, you will be contacted by phone and asked to pick your son up at the College. He will not return to the College until an interview is held between your son, yourselves, and myself.

At this interview the conditions upon which Ben will be readmitted to the College will be discussed. If the situation arises where it is deemed necessary to again suspend Ben from the College, your son's position here will be reviewed.

This letter is to be signed by you, the parents, Ben himself and returned.

If you wish to discuss this matter further, you may contact me at the College to make an appointment.

Deputy principal

On a brighter note I have included some of the poetry that I completed in Year Ten English. This shows my academic abilities about which my teachers so often reminded me, which I chose to ignore until I reached Year Twelve. The ironic thing is that I handed up lots of work I did in Year Ten again in Year Twelve because I was too lazy to do any new work. But I guess it doesn't matter because I did so well.

YOU DID THE RIGHT THING

I'm doing the right thing,
I think.
Good vs. Evil,
Bad against good.
I'm a freedom fighter,
I'm a baby killer,
I'm a murderer.
I'm trapped.
Drop a bomb on the Viet Cong,
Hope it hits,
Damn, I missed,
What was I thinking,
I must have been pissed,
I just killed a family of six.
Drop another and another,

Till good beats evil.
Bomb by bomb,
Spray by spray,
The nightmares are here to stay,
All I hear in my sleep,
Is the scream of the bombs,
That made so many people weep.
Too many men fell,
In the jungles of hell.
My mates are home,
But the scars are here to stay.
They said "Come on lads,
Come and help your country,
Come on, do what's right."

Remember, always look down,
Because if that's a mine,
Your legs are gone.
The noise the fright,
Will echo in your ears for life,
But remember lads,
You did what's right

STOP THE WAR!

Stop the war,
I can't handle it no more.
Good men dying,
Can't stop the mothers crying.

Fathers proud,
but nothing can stop the imminent mushroom cloud.
No winners in this amazing game of death and despair.
Where, where is my mate gone!
His wife Beth will soon be told of her love's bloody death.
Politicians sit in their chairs controlling us like pawns.
But do I see those bastards' legs being torn in two.
I think not, what a f*@#ing crock!
Some of these boys seem young enough to be back in their
    cots.
Stop the war, I can handle it no more.
Stop it now,
Because no one is going to stop that bullet
With your name on it!

KILL THE QUEEN

Kill the queen
and be ruled by Mr. Bean.
He'd do a better job
than that pompous snob.
He'd make us laugh
not like that silly old fart.
She can't run her kids
so what's going to happen to us.
She made a fuss when the stupid bag
fell out of a double decker bus.
She broke her hip in the fall
the media had a ball.
They said they cared
but all they wrote about
was her damn hair.
Get off the throne
and let's watch her moan.
No one likes
no one cares.
Let's assassinate this phoney
and her snobbish heirs.

Get her off the throne
get her off our money.
Get her out of the palace
for which we pay.
Don't throw flowers
throw grenades in vain
to cause maximum republican pain!

My report card from Year Ten is basically the same, with the same comments I have had since I was in prep—for example, "Ben has the ability to do well in this subject when he applies himself. He is often more interested in attracting attention for himself then concentrating on his work." I found some more interesting information. The subjects that I had an interest in, such as History, Geography, and English to a certain degree, I did exceptionally well. My grades indicate this. In History and Geography I got straight As but in subjects where I had no or little interest I failed. For example, in science and woodwork I didn't even hand one piece of work in.

It might be of interest to look at your own child's life. I bet you that your ADHD child does exceptionally well at things he enjoys or has an interest in. Conversely, when asked to do simple things like clean his room, it is nearly impossible. There is a very good reason for this. An ADHD child sees little benefit in doing something that he sees as boring. So the answer to this is to redirect these interests into the classroom. If he has to do a science project on coal production and he has the least interest in coal production, I can bet you that he won't do it or he will get a bad grade. But if he likes cars, why don't you speak to the teacher and ask him/her if he can do a research project on cars instead? Some people may say, "Well, that's not what we are studying." But I think it would be a lot more beneficial for your child to learn something rather than nothing. The good thing with this is that as your child gets older he can choose the subjects he wants to study, which allows this to happen a lot easier.

On a closing note, I loved every minute at that school and it holds some of my best experiences in life. Because the school only went to Year Ten once again my parents were on the hunt for another school. They found it, a new college, the same school that had rejected my plea to attend their school only a year before. But this time I got in. I never told them that I had already tried previously.

To finish up with Year Ten I have included the letter my teacher gave me on my last day. He gave the letters as awards with fitting names on them for each student. I won the award for the student who repeatedly tried to break every school rule and succeeded. This is the letter he wrote to me and it makes me feel good every time I read it.

Dear Ben,

Well, what can I say? You've certainly given me lots of material to talk about at dinner parties! Ben, even when you've been a complete pill and I've wanted to throttle you, I've still always cared about you. I think you are a really fantastic person and you have so much to give and offer. I have loved getting to know you and I think that there will be a definite emptiness in my class (it will also be quiet!)

Some of my fondest memories of this year have involved you—your fantastic poem on the Vietnam War; talking to you while you were in sick bay; sitting on the step of the staff house talking about having your operation on your legs, etc, all these things!

I hope that you can look back on your time here with happiness. I am certain that you could be a success at whatever you put your mind to. Aim high, Ben, and don't sell yourself short.

Be good!

Best wishes for a happy future

Homeroom Teacher

When I was younger I would read this letter to pick me up. I would also read the letter when I was being lazy at school and in life generally. I love the last line, "I am certain that you could be a success at whatever you put your mind to. Aim high, Ben and don't sell yourself short!" I just hope that I haven't sold myself short in life because I wouldn't like to let such a great person and friend down after everything he has done for me!

Thanks, from your good friend Ben Polis.

Co-educational college! Time to shape up or ship out!

Year Eleven was a real turning point in my life. Unlike most parents of boys at my old school, my parents thought it would be beneficial if I went to a different school in a different area. They thought my reputation as a troublemaker would not follow me to this school as well. This gave me the opportunity to put my future in my own hands. It was up to me now. I didn't have anyone else to blame if I didn't succeed to my abilities, which my previous teachers believed I had not used fully. It was a co-educational Catholic school.

My parents were a bit apprehensive about sending me to a co-educational school, believing that I would not be able to succeed with the distraction of females in my class. This thinking was due to the success that I had at an all-boys' school. However, this did not matter as much as my parents had anticipated. The reason for this was when I was at an all-boys school it was expected that we would act like a dick and fool around. Going to an all-boys' school is like going to school with your football team. All boys' schools allow a lot more leeway with boisterous behavior. I learned pretty quickly that attending a co-educational school is a totally different

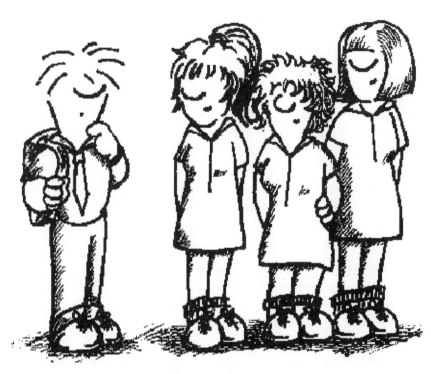

environment. At a co-educational school you can't act like a dick and play a fool because you make yourself look like a fool in front of the girls. This would not have been the case if I had attended a co-educational school in my younger years. People believe that you grow out of ADHD but that is not true. You just learn to control your behavior better as you mature. In theory this should have been the case but it was not. I still acted like the class clown because that's who I am. I will never change and I don't think I should have to change. If people don't like me I believe that's their problem.

When I first started at college it was not a big change. I made some friends pretty fast and I settled in pretty well. I still acted like a fool but the difference this time was that I wanted to succeed at my schoolwork. I remember the first time I handed in my first assignment. The teacher would not accept it. She didn't believe I had done it myself. At first I was really angry with this but I now understand why this was the case. I did no work in class; I called out constantly and didn't take any books to class. This was how I have always studied at school, by just listening to the teacher. I don't have the concentration to write things down and if I do I get bored and blank out. Well, I handed in a perfect piece of work and got an A for it. But my father had to write a letter to say I had done it. It was during Year Eleven that I really started to often use my self-help techniques. I guess I had always sort of used them but I had not used them enough to understand their true power.

Well, I passed Year Eleven with average grades. I did fail two subjects, Accounting and Physical Education, which seems pretty stupid considering that I should have excelled in these subjects. But again these subjects did not stimulate my interests and I deliberately failed them. You may be thinking, why would I deliberately fail these subjects? The reason was that I had completed three extra units in Year Ten doing two Year Eleven subjects. So my theory was that it didn't matter if I failed two subjects. This sounds dumb but this did let me pass my other subjects, which I was in danger of failing, anyway. My parents were furious with this decision I had made. My answer to this was: "It will be fine, it always is!" This became a bit of a catch phrase of mine when my parents were worried about my future. Again I was right and it was fine.

I did get suspended a couple of times in Year Eleven and had a number of after-school and Saturday detentions. These disciplinary actions were fueled by my disruptive behavior in class. But I was not fighting any more like I had before. I also found that my disruptive behavior in classes got worse as I got older. There is a very good reason for this, which I will discuss later.

Below is my Year Eleven report card:

COMMENTS FROM HOME ROOM TEACHER

Ben has settled well into the 11D homeroom and the calm and respectful atmosphere that we have developed. He is to be congratulated on his involvement in the co-curricular activities and for his co-operation in carrying out homeroom duties, including raffle ticket sales for Year Eleven Social Services causes. Ben is always courteous and well mannered. I look forward to witnessing and encouraging his continued academic development over the all-important second semester. Thanks for your support in homeroom, Ben. A very successful semester.

As you can see, my academic performance had improved considerably. But if I continued to get these grades they would not have got me into university. So once again I had to improve or I was going to be labeled a loser again. My first hurdle was to pass Year Twelve, which was no mean feat in itself. Well, the big year had arrived and it was sink or swim time again for me.

Year Twelve: Who would have thought I would have made it this far?

During Year Twelve I made some very radical changes in my life, which I have used ever since. These changes in both thinking and implementation I believe to be the determining factor which changed my life. I also feel they are an invaluable tool for your own child's schooling. I just wish I had discovered them earlier because my life would have been a lot easier. But I guess it doesn't matter.

Well, Year Twelve started and I had a point to prove to the world. I remember telling Mum, "I am going to show all those people who

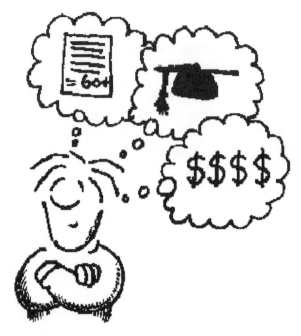

thought I was a loser!" I also remember writing down my goals at the start of Year Twelve, which were as follows:

> Pass Year Twelve without getting kicked out!
> Get a ENTER score over 60 (an ENTER score is the grade you get for doing Year Twelve. It is out of a possible 99).
> Get into university!
> Pass university!
> Make a million dollars before I am thirty!

BACKGROUND ON VCE PROCEDURES

VCE (Victorian Certificate of Education) is awarded to Year Twelve students who pass four nominated Year Twelve subjects.

These subjects are measured by three assignments during the year. Called CATS or (common assessment tasks), these CATS are around two thousand words each and take forever! You do one CAT in each semester, or half year. Along with this you do a number of minor work tasks that are not graded but you must pass them to get the VCE. So you do one CAT in semester one and then another in semester two. This is followed by an exam at the end of the year. The work load in Year Twelve is the hard thing about getting your VCE. So this means excellent organizational skills, which ADHD kids lack. But I had to be organized!

Semester one. Freak to geek in 17 years!

I was a new person. My parents could not believe their eyes. I was doing homework but not a little homework. I had become "The Homework Machine"—this was the name I called myself. The experts say that routine is vital for an ADHD child and even an adult and they are bloody right! Let me tell you my daily routine during Year Twelve.

Go to school and try to act cool. At school I was still Ben Polis. I still got kicked out of classes. I disrupted classes, walked out of classes and didn't go to classes. I don't know how many times during Year Twelve people asked me, "Are you passing?" "Yeah, of course!" I replied with a cheeky grin!

Go to after-school detention, get another detention for talking during my detention. Then do it all over again tomorrow.

Get the train home, give heaps to train passengers, buy two potato cakes from the fish and chip shop and walk home.

Watch television for about an hour. Turn television off at five o'clock.

Take two Ritalin.

Go down to my room. Then clean my room and my desk.

> Get a drink and some food to munch while doing homework so I don't use the excuse of being hungry to stop doing homework.
>
> Lock my door, turn on my stereo so I won't get bored.

By doing this I had created the perfect working environment for any student, but more importantly I had created the perfect working environment for an ADHD student.

Then I did the most amazing thing I have ever done in my life — I did homework and lots of it.

I would start doing homework at five o'clock and then stop at around eight o'clock to have dinner. But this is the most important thing that your child can learn from my routine. Once I had finished my dinner I would *run* back to my room and lock my door. Strange? Yes! But there is a very good reason for this. The reason I would run to my room was so I would not be distracted from anything else and stop doing my homework!

After dinner I would study till two o'clock in the morning—an incredible feat for any student but a miracle because I have ADHD. The amazing thing about this whole picture I am painting for you is that my medication had worn off. But I had captured my limited concentration and directed it to my schoolwork. This can only be done by me taking away all distractions.

Then I would go to sleep and do it all over again the next day.

I did do a lot of homework in Year Twelve but that was because I had to. Remember, I never did any work at school because I couldn't concentrate. A funny thing I found in Year Twelve concerned all my Year Twelve teachers. I was always being lectured to settle down at school and do more school work. But this all changed when I handed in my first round CATS in semester one.

I remember the day like it was yesterday. It was judgement day for me! I had not gone to school on that day and my mother had driven me to get my grades. I walked into school and I remember being so nervous. I received my grades from the Year Twelve office and busted the envelope open. All the other Year Twelves were doing the same. I yelled out at the top of my lungs, "*I got four As and one B+!*" Highlighting my impulsivity again! This was followed by loud laughter. I replied to this, "Nah, seriously, I got straight As!" Then people started to grab the piece of paper off me to look at my grades. Then they were even checking the name to see if it was mine. I then ran like a bat out of hell to show my mum. She didn't believe me either. What the hell is wrong with all these people? I couldn't believe how many people thought I was *dumb!*

The most important thing I learned from my first round CAT marks was that I had always thought and believed I could achieve at school but I had never ever proven myself. But now I had. I learned that if I applied myself I could achieve results far beyond my wildest dreams. I always believed that if you do something well and to your best ability anyone can achieve. However, I had never put this into practice. I always did things to the bare minimum to just pass. This theory I believe in is sort of like a religion I live by now. If I am going to do something it must be to the best of my abilities and if it is not I do not bother completing it. Along with this I also believe that if you get knocked down and don't succeed you must take that on board and try harder next time. As the saying goes, "Try, try, try again and you will succeed!"

My belief was tested by my father late one night. I was doing homework well past two o'clock. My father came into my room and asked me how I was going at school. I replied, "Everything is fine but I am sick of doing homework and I am tired and I want to go to bed." To my very upsetting surprise he told me that I was not doing enough homework and I wasted my time too much. He then told me that if I tried harder I would have got straight As and that the one B+ I got would have been an A if I wasn't so lazy and I tried harder. This made me so upset and angry. I told him to f*@# off and stop being so hard on me! I then told him that if this was

Adelaide (my sister) he would be the one doing her homework and she would be at the pub! My mother came downstairs because of the yelling between my father and I. She told him that he expected too much from me!

I was so upset because I wanted my parents to be proud of me and tell me they were proud of me. I knew they were proud of me but I could not believe what my father had told me. Looking back on it now, I understand what my father was really trying to get across. It wasn't that I had not tried enough or I was lazy. He just wanted me to do well and the only way he has ever known to do well and get ahead in life is to work harder than everyone else. So basically what he was saying was, "Ben, you must try harder and harder so you succeed." That's basically what I believe in today. He was right as usual, I guess. If I had tried harder I would have got straight As. I had reached my mental and physical boundaries and instead of stopping there, I should have pushed my boundaries until either they broke or I did. Sounds extreme but that's what I believe!

Semester two, the final hurdle!

Looking back on semester two now, it makes me quite angry. Not at the teachers or my parents or life in general. I get angry at myself. I had done really well in first semester but I did not achieve the same results in the next. They were not bad—they were quite good—but they could have been better and they should have been. I sort of lost my way during semester two. I still did all my homework but it was not at the same high standard as previously. I had had enough of school and I wanted to finish.

I did not put the same amount of effort into my CATS. Once I had achieved a level I believed would get me a good grade, that was good enough. I had sinned against my own religion. I had not

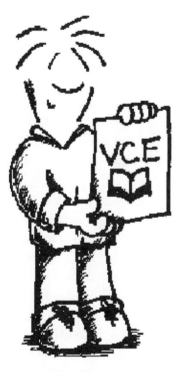

exceeded my boundaries—I had reached them and quit. I put this down to a couple of reasons. The first is I really started to hate school and I didn't want to go any more. I just wanted to sit at home and do my work from there. But this was not possible. Or was it? The second reason was that I was sick of doing meaningless school work that took up so much time and I didn't learn anything from it. I wanted to be at university now and learn about things I was interested in. These interests are basically business studies and the finer details of the economy. Some people hate these topics but they really get my mind stimulated, unlike English or Mathematics.

The third reason I hated being at school was pure boredom. I hated all my subjects except Economics. The work was mind-numbing rubbish. So, as in previous years, I resorted to disruptive behavior to relieve the boredom. I disrupted most of my classes by calling out and just being stupid. People kept asking me, "How can someone so smart be such a *fool?*" I told them how it is, I just like to muck around!

This question of my intelligence would again be highlighted by one of my teachers, when we had to start making decisions for preferences for university courses. I had my heart set on studying at Deakin University, doing a Bachelor of Business in commerce. I organized a meeting with her and told her what I wanted to study.

She told me that people like me didn't go to university! She thought it would be better if I did a TAFE course and then after I completed that I could apply for university, but at a lesser university. This made me so angry. I told her that I wanted to go to university and I was going to get into a good university. She then asked me in a very sarcastic tone what my grades were like for first semester. I told her, in the same sarcastic tone she had used, and her whole mood changed. I then decided I had got this far without anyone else's help so I was going to choose a university myself and that's what I did.

Well, this constant disruptive behavior of mine was not tolerated. I was constantly suspended and threatened with expulsion. This was a real issue that I had to deal with. I had made it so far but I was on the verge of expulsion. The coordinator had developed a plan, which would hopefully see me through the rest of the year. When I was feeling, or the teacher was feeling, I was going to lose it—what I mean by lose it is disruptive behavior—I was to leave the classroom and go to the library. Well, I loved this plan. It allowed me to self-medicate myself with self-imposed isolation as I did at home. The only problem was the library now had to contend with my disruptive behavior. The only flaw in the plan was that libraries and a disruptive ADHD student don't really work well, as you can imagine.

I got through the final semester but it was not an easy journey. I was expelled sort of but not as seriously as it could have been. The final exams were looming in around six weeks. By this time in the year I hated school even more than previously. I wanted out and I could not control my impulsive urges. I called out more and more and disrupted every class, including Economics. This was not tolerated by the school. The problem was it was the most important part of the year. All the students were cramming hard and really trying their hardest to study. But I had reached my limits and could not concentrate or be bothered to study. The school had had enough and told me that I was not to come back to school. The reason they gave was that I was constantly disrupting exam preparations. However, I was to come to school every couple of days and hand in work and receive work to do. Along with this, I was allowed to sit my exams at the college instead of doing them in the city. So I guess I was really lucky that I was allowed to do my exams and had not been expelled. On a brighter note though, this was just what I had wanted all along. This was perfect for me. It allowed me to finish off my assignments in time, which would have been harder if I had stayed at school.

Looking back on this now I wish I had stuck it out and controlled my erratic behavior a little better. The reason I feel this way is the marks I got in my final exams. By being at home I disadvantaged myself tremendously because I did not get the same level of exam preparation as everyone else. I did have the time to put in the study at home. But I was not in a mental state of mind to put in the hours required to pass the exams with flying colors. I had done enough work during the year to pass the exams well. But the marks I achieved in the second round of CATS and the exams underscored the predicament I had put myself in and the consequences of it.

I still did quite well considering I was not at school for the exam preparation. Most students would be pleased with these results. But I had sold myself short and I know that now but there is no point crying over spilled milk. The one thing I took out of my poor exam marks was exactly the same as my second round of CAT marks. I had done no study to achieve two B+s and three Bs in my exams, so who knows what I could have achieved if I had applied myself better? But it does not matter—I still made it to university.

So I finally had done it. I passed Year Twelve and received my VCE. It only took six schools, 5,000 detentions, 300 days of suspension and a case load of Ritalin. Passing Year Twelve would have to be one of my proudest moments. I had finally proven all the doubters wrong. I would love to go back to my Year Seven coordinator and wave my certificate in her face. It is teachers like that who do nothing for an ADHD student. Encouragement is the only way to get through to an ADHD student. It makes no sense constantly putting an ADHD student down because they will only start to believe what they are being told, that they are a troublesome burden on the school.

However, on a funny note, in Year Twelve there were some memorable moments that make me laugh. The first was putting the Year Twelve school captain in a wheelie bin and shutting the lid so she could not get out. It was good for a laugh even though it was at her expense.

The second incident I will always be remembered for. It was the last day of school which I was allowed to attend. The last day of school is known as change of ID day. Everyone dresses up as someone else. I had been thinking of who my identity would be for months. Then like a lightning bolt it hit me one day while I was getting yelled at by the director of students. I didn't like this man, and wanted to make him look stupid but just didn't know how.

Well, on the last day of school I remember him telling me before we all got changed that I had better be on my best behavior. I told him I would and that I had a little surprise for him. He didn't have a clue what I had been concocting for months. I got changed and walked outside as though nothing was different.

I then started to order students around. I couldn't believe it—I had made such a great uniform to look like this teacher people thought I was him. When everyone finally worked out it was me they were in hysterics. When this teacher came to say goodbye to Year Twelve he was greeted with further hysterical laughter, because I was imitating him behind his back. I walked up behind him and told him in his voice, "Tuck that shirt in or I will give you a detention, Ben Polis!" This was again followed by laughter. We had a photo taken together and I said, "How do you like your surprise?" He walked off and didn't come back. I had finally got the last laugh! It only took two years! This is definitely the best way to get back at a teacher you don't like. It provides years of pay-back when your classmates look back in their yearbook. So the moral to this story is do not mess with a creative ADHD child because you will come off second best.

Ben Polis is going to university! Yeah, right!

I did not get into Deakin University because I forgot to change my preferences. This again highlights my lack of organizational skills. Forgetting to change my course preferences was one of the most upsetting moments in my life. Now it was in the lap of the gods. The placements came out and I couldn't believe it. I got into a more preferred business university than I had ever imagined. I scored a TER (tertiary entry score) of 78.05 out of a possible 99.5, which is a good score. This also again proved my ability when I had written down that I wanted a TER above 60 in my goals at the start of the year. The problem was that to study most business courses I needed above 81, which I did not get. It was such a nervous time in my life because I knew that if I had tried as hard as I had in first semester I would have got around 85 and easily got into any course. But again luck was on my side. I was accepted into the School of Business at RMIT in the undergraduate Bachelor of Business in Administration. The reason I say luck was on my side again was that you needed a TER of around 93, which I was nowhere near. I was the last person to be let into the course and I

got the lowest TER. I couldn't believe it. I have always felt that I have been lucky and that someone is always looking out for me. I don't know who it is but thanks, whoever you are.

So I had finally achieved my personal goal. I was going to university and I had achieved all this with a learning disability. I would like to know what that learning disability is because I haven't worked out what it is yet. I have often wondered what my life would be like if I didn't have ADHD and I don't think it would as successful as it is today. I like to think of myself as one of the lucky people who has ADHD because I feel that I wouldn't be as intelligent if I didn't have ADHD.

The greatest thing about university is not the actual study at university. The thing I love the most is when I see people on the train who I once went to school with in my younger years and they ask me where I am going. I love the reaction I get when I tell them I am going to university. I always had such a motivational problem when I had to go to school but when I get up for university I wake up with a smile on my face. Every day I go to university it is a reminder of how far I have come. You may think this sounds a bit conceited, but I am damn proud that I am at university and I can't wait for the day my name is called out and I receive my degree at graduation. I have pictured this day over and over again in my head and it gets better every time.

University is the place to be if you have ADHD!

University is definitely the place for me. My Year Ten English teacher told me one day that I would be more suited to university than high school. I never really understood this until I got there. The reason university is so good for an ADHD student is the learning style that they use.

The first thing I realized when I went to university was that acting like a fool is not tolerated as in high school. It is not that they don't allow it. It is that you choose to be there and if you act like a fool what the hell are you doing there in the first place? You are there because you want to be there and you want to do well, not for your parents but for yourself. If you do not apply yourself to your highest abilities the only person you are letting down is yourself.

The second reason university is the place for an ADHD student is that you go to university and you sit in a lecture for a couple of hours and use all your concentration on listening. Then you have a break for an hour or two, which lets you rejuvenate your concentration stores and then you have a tutorial for around an hour. Then you go home and study in your own learning style. This learning is not possible in high school because you are locked up for hours on end with many distractions. Along with this, when you are at university if you feel that you cannot concentrate and you need a break before the next class you can just walk out any time. Conversely at high school if you walked out of a class you would receive a detention.

The third reason university is the place to be if you have ADHD is that you have chosen the course you are doing. We all know that ADHD people have interests and often hyper-focus on these topics. So if you choose a course that you are interested in you can direct this hyper-focus into your course and achieve tremendously. But the key to this success is to choose a course that you are truly interested in. I know if I had chosen to do Accounting because I would have been paid well at the end of it I would have failed it. The reason is I cannot concentrate on things that I am not interested in. So instead of using this as a disadvantage you should, as I have, turn it around and use it as an advantage.

There is one thing you must be very careful of when your child goes to university. The ordered routine of high school is not prevalent at university. You do not have to go to class or even hand in work. You do not have a teacher yelling at you to hand in an assignment—it is up to you. Along with this when you first go to university you are not told anything—you have to work out everything yourself. This is a recipe for disaster for an ADHD student. To counter this problem I advise that you or your child find out as much information as possible about the university beforehand. Find out where your course office is and where you hand in your assignments. Along with this keep a diary of all due dates and be extremely organized. I also advise that you get the numbers of all your lecturers before you start the course. This will allow you to find out answers to questions concerning your course when they arise. The most important thing an ADHD student should do before attending university is to locate the library. This may seem stupid, especially in my case because I hate libraries, but libraries can be an ADHD student's best friend. Libraries provide the perfect working environment for an ADHD student because they are quiet and you can isolate yourself, allowing you to capture your limited concentration. Another service university often provides is learning aids. You can receive extended time on your exams and even get scribes to write down notes. I have not used any of these but they would be of benefit. But I do not want to stand out and look different.

Well, I achieved good results in my first year at university and was quite happy with my course. But while I was handing in an assignment I saw a poster for a new course. It was a Bachelor of Business in Entrepreneurial Studies and I was immediately interested. I found out a bit more about the course and I applied. The course was designed for students who had a good business idea or were already running their own business. I didn't have a business but I had lots of good ideas. I had an interview and I could feel it was not going so well until I decided that I would again use my ADHD as an advantage. I had already started writing this book but didn't want anyone to know. I told the interviewer what I was doing and how I was helping other kids who suffer from ADHD. She was pretty impressed and I knew that I had got in.

So that's what I am doing now. I have been doing this new course for around six weeks and I love it. It allows me to express all my weird and wacky ADHD ideas without narrow-minded people knocking them as they did in the past. I guess only time will tell if these ideas of mine will be successful. But I believe if I try hard enough and push myself they will succeed.

Well, that's my life. There are many things I am not proud of and some things I am extremely proud of. I just hope that I have provided a more positive outlook on ADHD. I was a very upset and angry child in my younger years. But now I could not be happier and I would not change a thing in my life because I feel that I have learned a lot from my experiences and that I can teach other people as a result of them. I remember one day only a couple of months ago at work when someone asked me, "What are you so happy about?" I replied, "Life in general!"

Strategies to success!

I feel strategies are the most fundamentally useful tool to overcome and use ADHD to your advantage. Some elite ADHD doctors will dispute this statement. They believe that medication is the only way to treat ADHD. I am not a critic of medication because I use it nearly every day, but only when I need it. The argument I put forward about medication is quite simple. Medication does not stop but only limits the impulsive urges to which ADHD children and even adults are prone. An example of this is if your son is on medication and his brain tells him to jump from a tree. No medication is going to stop this thought process. Therefore you must teach your son to think about the consequences of jumping from the tree. I use a technique of deciphering which is a good thought and which is not such a good thought. I often put myself in other people's shoes and wonder whether if I were someone else, would they jump from the tree? This allows me to decide between a good thought and a bad thought. The argument I often get when I put this technique forward is when a person says that their son would not be able to think about that before he jumps because he is too impulsive. This is often true. But if you drill this into your son every day he will eventually remember when he is doing something abnormal. People often say that ADHD kids don't think before they do something. But I disagree with that theory.

ADHD kids do think before they do something but they do not think about the consequences after the action. As you know, every action has a reaction but ADHD kids often forget this.

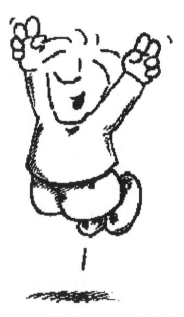

Why are ADHD children prone to anger, violence and erratic behavior?

Parents often ask why their child is so angry and violent. Some people think these are symptoms of ADHD. But this is not true. I have severe ADHD and I was an extremely angry and violent person. But as I grew up I had no reason to be angry and violent and bash innocent people and my family. So, you ask, why are ADHD children so angry and violent? It is not a *symptom* of ADHD but a *result* of ADHD. To understand why your child is so angry, upset and violent you must understand the world your child lives in. People who do not have ADHD really don't understand what it is like to have ADHD and therefore they do not understand how to deal with it and control it. So I will try to explain to you what it is like to have ADHD so you can better understand your own child.

What is it really like to have ADHD?

ADHD is often classified as a disorder that affects concentration, usually associated with naughty or just bad children. This is a common belief of people who do not understand ADHD and the media subsequently reinforces this. ADHD children are often

ـjust bad kids because of these erratic behavioral and
ـial patterns. But ADHD goes much further than this. To
understand what I am about to say you must look at it from your
child's point of view and not from your normal perspective.

Have you ever done something and afterwards wondered, "Why
the hell did I do that or say that?" That is exactly what it is like to
have ADHD. But the only problem is you don't understand why
you did that because in your mind that is what your brain told you
to do or say.

An example of this I often use is: If a normal person's brain tells
them "I am hungry so feed me," what do you do? You feed yourself
by making a sandwich or something. This seems normal to you,
because your brain told you that you were hungry so you did it.

Now let's look at it from an ADHD perspective. You are sitting
down watching television and just relaxing. You still have the same
thought. "I am hungry, so feed me." So what do you do? You get
up to feed yourself. You are out of your seat and running to the
kitchen. But then you forget why you were getting a sandwich. But
as you are running to the kitchen you see the dog sitting on the
carpet. Then your brain tells you to kick the dog just like your brain
told you to make a sandwich. Then the dog bites you and you kick
it again. The dog runs off and you wonder why the dog bit you. But
then your brain tells you that you're still hungry so you make a
sandwich. But just before you make a sandwich your mum yells at
you and smacks you for kicking the dog. But you're wondering
what your mum smacked you for because you were just making a
sandwich. Then you go mental and start to kick your mum and tell
her that she is a *cow!* But you don't realize that you just called your
mum a cow because you just wanted to make a sandwich. Then you
go back and continue watching television.

Now look at it from a mother's perspective. How the tables turn.
My son was running to the kitchen, kicked the dog, the dog bit my

son, my son then kicked the dog again and the dog ran off. So I smacked my son for kicking the dog. Then my son hit me back and called me a *cow*. Then he sat down and continued watching television as if nothing had happened.

The mother then starts to cry because she can't understand what is wrong with her son. She asks herself, "Why did my son call me a *cow* and hit me?" She then thinks to herself, "Maybe I am just a bad mother." Then depression sets in and the mother just can't handle it any more.

Another example of how your son's thought process works is by looking at yours. You are going shopping and a large woman walks past and knocks you with her stomach. You think to yourself, "Watch what you're doing, fatty!"

Now look at it from your son's perspective. You are going shopping but you really hate shopping and want to be watching television. You are already in a bad mood because your mum won't take you to the toy shop. So you are walking along insulting your mum because she won't take you to the toy shop. You are so angry you are going to explode. Then a large woman walks past and knocks you with her stomach. You turn around and yell at the top of your lungs, "Stupid fat bitch, watch where you wave that thing, you're so fat your stomach has its own postcode!" Then your mum smacks you because some fat lady knocked you.

Looking at this from your mum's perspective, you are the one at fault. She is crying inside, asking herself "Why can't he just keep his mouth shut?" Looking at it from your perspective, you think it's your mum's fault because if she had just taken you to the toy shop none of this would have happened—and the fat bitch deserved it.

What makes an ADHD child angry and violent?

We all know that ADHD children are often extremely violent, especially towards their family. Parents often do not understand why their child expresses violence towards the people they love but at the same time does not vent this anger on other people. This creates the belief in parents that they are the cause of their child's anger and that they must be at fault. To understand this and therefore correct the problem, parents must again take a snapshot of their child's life.

Normal children attend school with few obstacles. But an ADHD child is faced with huge obstacles every day. At such a young age these obstacles seem to be like crossing the English Channel. To understand this concept I will again describe your child's world. I like to use an example of a volcano to describe ADHD anger. Anger builds up like a lava in a volcano until it reaches such a point it explodes. But this is where parents often get confused. They do not understand why something as trivial as brushing your teeth can trigger such an angry outburst. This is when the volcano example comes into it. But the best thing about the volcano example is that like volcanos you can gauge when and where they are going to explode. You, too, can measure and predict when and where one of these outbursts is going to happen. But unlike volcanos you can also slowly release pressure so they do not build up and cause widespread destruction.

The volcano example

Your son wakes up in the morning tired after only a couple of hours' sleep. You think to yourself, "How can he be so tired? I put him to sleep early." Many people don't realize the difficulty that ADHD people have in getting to sleep. It's not that they are not tired—they are often exhausted after such an energetic day. They just can't get to sleep because unlike normal people whose mind stops when they go to bed, an ADHD person's mind never stops. Stimulant medication such as Ritalin also causes insomnia. So your son wakes up tired and has to face another day of obstacles. He wakes up in a bad mood and then has to go to school. The first level of lava has been placed in the volcano without even realizing it.

When he finally gets to school after many frantic minutes in the morning he is placed in a restricted environment. The class is told to open their books. But your son does not hear this command because he is not concentrating. Again, this is another untrue common belief—that ADHD kids don't concentrate. Your son is not concentrating on the teacher but on something else that he finds more mentally stimulating. His concentration has already been sapped due to lack of sleep. He is then told off for not opening his book, but he can't understand why he is being told off again because he didn't remember being told to open his book. He is now getting even more confused in this environment, especially if he lacks academic skills. He sees the rest of the students doing work but he can't do it, and he doesn't understand why. The second level of lava has been placed in the volcano of anger.

It's time for lunch but your son has to stay back, either to finish his work or for some misdemeanor. He looks out at the other kids playing and thinks to himself, "Why am *I* not playing outside?"

However, now he is the only one in the classroom and he can now finish his work because he has created the perfect working environment. But he still can't understand why he couldn't do it before. He thinks to himself, "Why am I so different to the other kids?" The third layer of lava has been laid.

Lunch is over but your son has had no time to burn off any of his extra energy or frustration. He now has to go back to class and do more unstimulating schoolwork. He sees his mate next to him making a paper aeroplane. He thinks to himself, "That seems more interesting than doing math," so he makes one. But he makes his aeroplane bigger and better than his mate's. This is where ADHD kids just don't understand the concept of being subtle. Your son has become so interested in making his aeroplane that he is in a totally different world. This is referred to as hyper-focusing, to which ADHD people are prone. He now wants to test his plane and he throws it across the classroom. It hits a girl in the head and he is sent outside. While sitting outside he thinks to himself, "Why does everyone pick on me so much? My friend was also making a paper aeroplane but he didn't get in trouble."

This is where ADHD kids suffer the most. They don't really understand how distracting or over the top their behavior is because it seems so normal to them. The fourth level of lava has been laid in the volcano of anger.

You pick up your son and he seems really happy. You believe he is happy because he had a good day at school. But really he is so happy because he is out of school and in the sanctuary of people who love him and don't treat him differently. Your son goes home and throws his bag on the floor right in the way of everyone. He sits himself down and watches television for hours and hours. You think he is just being lazy but he is not. I will explain this later.

It's now time to do homework. But you know and he knows that it is not going to happen without a fight. You turn the television off and you have successfully triggered off the volcano of anger. But you are thinking, "What the hell did I do that was so bad? I just turned the television off." Your son then goes into a rage of anger, yelling and swearing at you. But you're not at fault, you're just the lava field where your son can release the anger built up over the day.

There are a couple of things you must realize when your son goes off like this. The first is that when your son works himself up into these fits of anger he does not know what he is doing. He is so angry, and when he explodes he does not understand what he is doing or saying. He may punch you and kick you but he honestly does not know what he is doing. This seems really strange to normal people but it is true. The thing about these outbursts is that they can last only a couple of minutes or maybe an hour. But afterwards he can be as nice as pie and settled and calm.

Normal people will see this as a total disregard for their behavior. But what makes it even worse is that parents will punish their child after he has released his anger. Then the whole circle starts off again. Your son does not know why he has now been sent to his room because he can't even remember punching and kicking you—subsequently laying the first layer of lava again.

People often ask me why it is the parents who receive the raw end of the violence. It's not that your son hates you and doesn't love you. It is the exact opposite. He does love you and that's why he does it. It sounds strange but that's what happens. He knows that if he explodes like this you will be there tomorrow and still love him. You are your child's lava field and like lava fields they are used over and over again to release the pressure.

What to do if you have an angry and violent ADHD child!

Violence can destroy any family but it makes it so much harder to handle when you love the violent person unconditionally. My parents once described me as an uncontrollable child, which is quite true. But what they didn't realize was that I couldn't control my own actions. So I guess they had no chance! It took me many years to understand why I was so angry and violent. But when I did, my whole life changed and so did my parents'. The thing about anger is it builds up until it explodes and then people you love get hurt. But there is an answer and a way to control anger, which I learned.

I have already outlined why ADHD kids are so angry but I

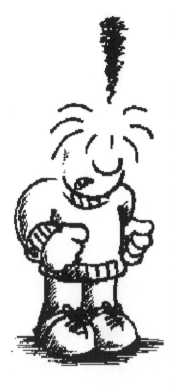

haven't told you what you really want to know. How do I stop it?

The answer to anger reduction is a long and hard journey but when you reach the end of that journey it is worth every step. The first thing you must do is understand why your son is angry. This can be mistaken for the incident that caused the violent explosion. But you must look beyond that and see into your son's world. His social environment is often the cause of most anger. The answer is to change it. The only way to do so is to build up your son's confidence so he believes he can take on the world. Most people don't know what it is like to be constantly put down every day for things that they think are normal, to be told that you're a bad kid and just plain dumb.

Building self-confidence can be done only by either of two things. The first is academic performance. But the problem again arises, "How can you teach an ADHD kid who doesn't want to learn?" This is a question I often get from parents. They say it sounds good in theory but the implementation is nearly impossible. I totally agree with this but there is an answer. The problem is that ADHD kids learn differently than normal kids. The learning system employed by schools is like teaching your child in another language. But there is an answer to this and I will discuss how to teach your child later.

The second way is to build confidence by sports or drama, etc. We all know that ADHD kids are very energetic. They often excel on the sporting field but the problem is that they have little confidence in themselves to do well. The other problem is that sports are often team sports and ADHD kids have trouble with social interaction. If sports and school work are not implemented properly they can be counter-productive.

When using sports to build confidence I suggest individual sports. This allows your son to develop a sense of responsibility for his actions. It also creates a sense of personal achievement lacking in team sports. How many coaches do you think are going to like a low-concentration threshold player when trying to give orders or plays? I know—not many. Even if your son is not good at his individual sport I suggest that you speak to his coach. If he never wins, who really cares? It's all about building confidence. You should tell your son's coach of his condition and then tell the coach how to help. Even giving your son an encouragement award would be extremely beneficial.

Once you have built your son's confidence up it's time to now mold him into a more settled person. I have already told you that your son cannot be responsible for his actions because he does not understand what he is doing wrong. I bet you that you have yelled at your son over and over again and it seems as though he is not listening. Well, you are right. You can yell at an ADHD child for hours and hours and he won't hear you because ADHD people have this uncanny knack of shutting the outside world off from themselves. *To get through to an ADHD child throw all normal disciplinary actions out the window.*

To really reduce anger, you must show your son what he is doing wrong when he is acting like this. ADHD children are very visual and experience most things through their eyes. So you tell me, what is the use of yelling at him at the top of your lungs? To get through to an ADHD child you must show him exactly what he is doing *at the time*. Not afterwards, not even ten minutes later. As soon as he does something you must show him what he is doing or he will just forget and the whole disciplinary action is useless.

The video camera and a simple tape recorder can be a parent's best friends. If your child is throwing a temper tantrum I suggest that you record it and play it back to him as soon as possible. Lock the child in a room and make them watch it over and over again until they realize what they have done and said. But don't let them out of their room until they have told you exactly what they have done wrong. This can be a life-changing moment for ADHD children because they finally see what they are doing wrong. The greatest thing about this tactic is that the next time your child goes crazy, all you need to do is to get out the video camera again. This visual cue tells them that they are acting as they did the last time they watched the video.

When your son has calmed down, I suggest that you sit him down and make him a sandwich and a drink and tell him that you love him. Your son is acting like this because his world is so hard to live in. He feels isolated, different and unloved. By showing him that you care for him instead of yelling at him and reinforcing his self-doubt, you are making him feel better about himself.

I also suggest that when your son does go mental you should let him go. Don't stop him or try to restrain him unless he is breaking things or endangering himself or other people. Your son has to release the volcano of anger and if he doesn't it will only build up more and more.

You can also try to predict when and where one of these violent outbursts is going to happen. Certain things trigger off these outbursts. I have learned that when I do not let off steam I often let it off on other people. By recording the dates, time and the circumstances of the outburst you can better predict future ones. If a pattern emerges, you can counter this by deliberately releasing anger in short bursts, for example, playing catch or having a kick of a football and so on.

The secret to releasing the volcano is to learn to live with it and not to restrain it. Your son must release this anger in short controlled bursts. One of the boys I tutor is quite violent at school, like I was. One day when I was trying to tutor him I was getting nowhere. I could see he was angry and just wanted to explode. So I decided that if he was going to explode the best person to vent his anger at would be me. I took him outside and we had the biggest fight—it lasted about forty minutes. His mother came outside and could not believe her eyes. Her son was kicking me, biting me, punching me and pulling my hair. His eyes were lit up and he looked mad! Most people would have been scared, but I knew exactly what he was going through. It wasn't that he hated me, because he loves me dearly, it was just that he had to release his anger. It's pretty hard to explain this to parents because it seems so wrong. It's like I am encouraging him to be violent. But what I was doing was allowing him to release his anger on me so that he would not release it at school, where he gets into trouble.

The only problem is it teaches him that violence solves things. So, afterwards, I lay next to him on the ground and we looked up at the sky for about fifteen minutes. I then explained to him that he couldn't act like this towards other people because they don't understand how much fun it is. After this, we did his homework. We had never had such a productive day of homework. This was due to him freeing his mind of anger and hate for the world, and especially schoolwork.

The other problem is that I don't know how many mothers like to have their hair pulled. None, I suspect. I then thought about this a little more. Then it hit me. Martial arts do three great things for ADHD kids. The first is that it allows them an outlet to release anger in a controlled environment. The second is that it teaches them to understand when and where they can use their fighting skills. Hopefully not on their sister. The third is it creates further self-esteem because they receive colored belts for their achievements.

The last thing I would like to mention about anger is that you must address it with an open mind. Sometimes you must condemn it and sometimes you have to encourage it. The thing about controlled anger is it teaches your child to control it when they feel as if they are going to explode. My mum often says, "Go for a run on the beach and let your aggro out." It works!

Where does ADD come from?

Only recently has this topic interested me and even excited me. The question many parents want to know is: Where does ADD come from—what causes ADD? We now know that it is hereditary and often comes from the father, but not in all cases. My interest has recently been fueled by a talk I attended in Australia by Thom Hartmann. His talk and discussion on ADD explained and reinforced what I already believed about ADD and the things I have discussed. I have often said things in my book that have no scientific backing, because I have told you just what I believe and why I believe it. Finally, I can explain things in a more scientific and credible manner. This theory of Hartmann's is only a theory but I honestly believe that it is the best theory of ADD I have heard. Most of the following is not my own work or theory but a reinterpretation of Thom Hartmann's work, which he has given me permission to do. You can read more on this in his excellent book, *Attention Deficit Disorder—A Different Perception*.

The hunter

In the medical field, Attention Deficit Disorder is labeled, as the

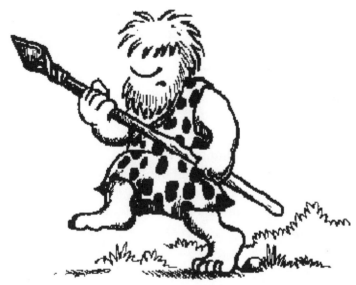

name suggests, a disorder or a deficit. However, I have a real issue, as do a lot of other people, with calling it a disorder. The reason I don't like it is that studies show that in some cases ADD affects approximately 20 per cent of the male population. I personally find it hard to believe that a disorder such as this can suddenly appear as it seems it has in the past twenty years. The answer is that it hasn't just appeared, it has always been there but has only come to the surface as a result of changes in our society. Let me explain how and why it has surfaced in such large numbers.

If you take a look at human society and its demographics over the past ten thousand years you will see a separation of two significant cultures and groups. The first group is the hunting society and it has many of the ADD traits we see today in our children and even in adults. To understand this, we must have a look at society and the lifestyle of the hunter.

What makes a good hunter?

What characteristics and personality traits did a hunter need to survive in his environment? Well, let me tell you, the same personality and character traits that ADD people have today. However, these traits are not often encouraged in our society, as they would have been in a hunting society.

Personality traits of a hunter!

Alertness and a sense of their environment

To be a successful hunter, you must be aware of your surroundings. When a hunter is on the hunt looking and searching for his next meal he must be constantly scanning his environment. If he does not have this personality trait it would make it impossible to find and kill his prey. If he is not aware when walking through the forest/jungle and does not notice a noise or get a glimpse of his prey, he could end up dead as a result of his lack of alertness.

When you compare this personality trait to our children you can see a direct link. We all know how much ADD children notice the smallest detail of things. It could be a spider walking up the wall or a bird's nest outside. ADD children are always being told to mind their own business. They are always wanting to know everything about everyone and everything. Parents are often bombarded with questions such as: "Why? How come? Can I touch it? Let me see?" etc. This becomes very annoying after a while but it is in their personality to be inquisitive. The upside to this personality trait is that they often have an excellent general knowledge. I have had some really good discussions with ADD kids that I could not have had with a non-ADD child.

However, this trait is not encouraged in our schooling system. Children are told what to do, and that's it. If they notice something interesting or a flaw in what the teacher is saying, they are told off. This really affects an ADD child because it comes so naturally to them.

Now! There is no tomorrow!

Another characteristic of a good hunter is his ability to disregard time and concentrate solely on the moment. When the hunt is on there is nothing else going on in his mind. All his concentration is on the hunt and nothing will take him away from that. Hunters live for the moment—they do not worry or care about what may be around the next tree or valley. If time were relevant to a hunter, it would be deadly. Can you imagine a hunter chasing his prey, then looking up at the sun, then thinking to himself, "Hey, I have been working hard, I should take a break." If this were the case, his meal would be long gone. Therefore, time must have no relevance and the only thing that matters is what is happening now.

ADD people of today have the same trait. Time is always a big problem with ADD people. They are always disorganized and late for appointments. ADD people have no sense of time and also live for the moment. If you were to follow an ADD person around for a day, you would notice something that normal people would think strange. Like a hunter, ADD people work in short hard bursts, which is then followed by nothing. They mope around the house until they find something they are interested in. Then the hunt is now on. They throw themselves into their work with incredible concentration. You yourself have most probably seen this with your own child. Your child will be doing something or focusing on something and seem to be mesmerised by it. You can call their name over and over again with no response. You pull them away from it, then they get free and start to stare at it again.

Time having no relevance is even more interesting when you look at older people with ADD. ADD adults often find themselves starting things in the middle of the night and working for hours and hours. They have totally disregarded time as a result of completely immersing themselves in the moment. This is also known as hyperfocusing. If we take a look at the working habits of Albert

Einstein, he would constantly immerse himself in his work and have no contact with other people until he was done. This is just another example of an ADD person hyperfocusing or throwing himself into the hunt.

Changing strategy at a moment's notice

A good hunter must be able to change his strategy at a moment's notice. If he is chasing one single animal and a herd of buffalo is spotted, he must make a quick decision. Does he keep hunting a single animal that is closer but not as big and therefore less valuable, or does he change his strategy and hunt the buffalo? The problem that a normal person would have in this scenario would be that they would first think about it and then act. But the opportunity would then be gone. Therefore impulsiveness is a must for a hunter.

In today's society, impulsiveness and quick decision-making can end in disaster. However, it is often vital in business. Many well-known entrepreneurs are suspected of having ADD. The argument against changing strategy and using impulsiveness is that they take risks and do not plan. This is very true. In business, you must have a plan for the future and you can't keep changing your business strategy every two weeks. But what makes these entrepreneurs different than normal people? It is their ability to change strategy at a moment's notice when the market demands it. In the same way, a hunter can quickly change his strategy in the hunt. Jumping from one idea to another is often a trait in ADD people. It is this ability to change their strategy or plan at a moment's notice that can either make or break an ADD person. If an ADD person learns to use their impulsiveness and control it, they can do incredible things. Conversely, it is also this impulsiveness and jumping from idea to idea that can make an ADD person's life harder than it needs to be.

Hunters think visually

Hunters think and experience things through seeing and visualizing things. Hunters have used pictures, symbols and paintings to communicate for thousands of years. The same is true for ADD people today. They would much rather see something and visually experience it than just read about it. This is a problem when it comes to reading. If a book does not describe visual objects, places and people, etc, it does not provide the visual stimulation needed to keep concentration. I once read about a famous inventor suspected of having ADD who would visualize all the cogs and moving parts in his mind before he even drew up the blueprints. Using visual stimulation for educational purposes is very helpful for younger ADD children.

Hunters thrive on the excitement of the hunt

Hunters thrive and become alive in the hunt. Conversely, they do not do as well at mundane and boring tasks. This can be seen clearly in ADD people. ADD children hate doing boring things such as homework and cleaning their room. They are labeled as lazy because they seem to do nothing. But when something excites and interests them they become alive and hyperactive, just like hunters do. The same goes for entrepreneurs in today's society. Why do all these entrepreneurs do crazy things and risk their life flying around the world in hot air balloons, flying a helicopter solo around the world and paying to go into space? I am not suggesting that all these men have ADD, but why do they do it? The simple reason is that they thrive on a challenge and, more importantly, the excitement. It's just like adrenalin junkies who jump off buildings and bridges. To get their next fix, they must do something more extreme than last time. ADD people are exactly the same. They are always hunting for excitement to satisfy their boredom.

High expectations of themselves and others

Hunters are very hard on themselves and others they work with in order to survive. If one member of the tribe lets them down while on the hunt it could mean death for one of the tribe members. When your life depends on split-second decision-making, to survive you tend to be very impatient and have a low frustration level.

In today's society where we must wait every day for something, ADD people seem to go crazy. Alexander Bell, who invented the telephone, is one of many inventors believed to have had ADD. But if he had imagined that it would cause his fellow ADD people so much frustration he would most probably not have invented it. It is funny watching an ADD person being put on hold on the telephone. Their face says it all! It's the same with bank lines. ADD people just want to do everything right away and when it takes too long they want to explode. Frustration and impatience can often trigger other less desirable traits in ADD people. This is especially the case in business. ADD people are often described as arrogant and abrupt. This is true, because like the hunter ADD people can't stand incompetence and people letting them down.

Normal people—steady as she goes

As I have explained, ADD is the remnants of necessary skills or personality traits needed to survive as a hunter. Therefore the question remains—where do normal people or non-ADD people originate? The theory states that the second society of primitive man is the agricultural society that then developed. Once again, we must look at what makes a good farmer. I bet you can guess that it's not any of the traits of a hunter.

What skills does a good farmer need?

Not easily distracted by his environment

A farmer must stay on task and not be distracted by his environment. Crops must be planted at certain times of the year. If farmers were easily distracted, as hunters can be, and decided to wander through the jungle to investigate a noise or fire, away from the village for days even weeks, by the time they returned, their window of opportunity to plant the crop would be gone and they would starve.

Slow and steady

A good farmer must put in a sustained effort over long periods of time. Conversely, a hunter must put in short bursts of energy to capture his prey. If a farmer put in high levels of energetic activity in short bursts, he would burn himself out. Could you imagine a farmer putting the same level of activity needed to catch a deer or a buffalo into harvesting? He would die. Therefore, slow and steady is the only way a good farmer can survive.

Plan for the future

Farmers are unlike hunters, who cannot foresee the future or do not care because they will deal with it when it arises. Farmers must and do plan for the future. If a farmer decided that he was sick of eating grain and planted a different crop that drained the nutrients from the soil but tasted better, he would starve in years to come. The same goes for planning for the winter months. Farmers must plan how much food can be eaten every day of the year. Their food supply must last all year round. Conversely, if a hunter were distributing the food, it would all be gone by winter, because hunters have trouble foreseeing and planning for the future.

Not easily bored

Farmers are not easily bored and do not have a problem with doing the same mundane tasks every day. Hartmann said that this is the nature of farming, a slow and sustained effort over long periods of time. When the crops have been planted or harvested, farmers find things to do—make new tools, furniture, barns, etc.

Cautious and patient

Farmers do not like risk because risk means danger, unlike a hunter, who must take risks to survive. It is not very dangerous planting a crop. But if the farmer does not plant the right crop, it can be disastrous to his whole community. Farmers do not face short-term danger like a hunter but can face long-term risk. Therefore, farmers are better organizers and plan for the future.

The nature of farming is patience, both with crops but more importantly with other co-workers, unlike hunters, who want everything now and can't wait for anything. If a hunter were placed into one of these primitive agricultural societies and asked to watch the crop grow, he would go crazy from boredom. It is just the nature of being a hunter.

What would happen if you put a hunter into a farming society?

Well, we have, and there are millions of these people throughout the world. But instead of calling them hunters we have labeled these people as suffering from Attention Deficit Disorder. The question arises—why there aren't equal numbers of farmers and hunters in today's society? The answer to this is that farming communities have evolved into large and powerful predominantly western countries or regions. Therefore hunting is no longer needed as a vital food source. Basically, the farmers took over the world and the hunting traits were lost forever. Or were they? The answer is *no!* The personality traits of primitive hunters are still alive today and it can be seen every day in your child.

However, the problem still remains. ADD people must live and survive in a predominantly farmers' world. This is why I feel that ADD has surfaced in such magnitude in today's society and especially in the past twenty years. Take a look at our school system. The modern school system is derived from the German school system created in the 1800s. In short, our school system discourages creative thinking and pushing the envelope. The current school system works very well for non-ADD types or farmers, because it was designed for that type of person—meaning repetitive, boring, disciplined, conforming, methodical and narrow-minded thinking.

Conversely, it does not work for an ADD or hunter type, who is punished for being creative, thinking outside of the square, being inventive, demanding, exciting, impulsive and asking the tough questions. Teachers do not know how to deal with these types of children. They have not been taught to teach hunters, only farmers. They only know how to teach the three Rs over and over again. And these teachers wonder why their ADD students are disruptive?

If I had been born forty years ago I would not be able to read or write. I say this because forty years ago the expectation to finish school and go to university/college was not voiced by society. I would have dropped out and got myself an apprenticeship after failing at school and being labeled just a bad kid or even stupid. I would have hated this because I would have found myself doing the same thing over and over again, which I can't stand. I would not have been detected as having ADD or minimal brain dysfunction, as it was called then. I would have most probably drifted from job to job, city to city, pub to pub. I would have been labeled as a drifter or even a loser. But I was not born forty years ago and I had to succeed in school because society expected it and therefore my parents and I subsequently did. However, this is definitely a key reason for the increase in ADD in recent years. I had to stay in school and succeed. If I hadn't, I would have found it very hard in life. Humans have always had learning disabilities but our society today places such an emphasis on education that the learning problems that some humans have must be addressed.

Another issue that is not often mentioned about the change in society is the role of the mother. During the 1960s the women's rights movement started to gather momentum. The liberation felt by women across the world subsequently changed society and the family culture. Women had been expected to stay at home and look after the children. However, as the woman's rights movement evolved, women started to enter the workforce. Today, it is normal for women to work and advance their careers. However, I personally believe this may be a reason why ADD has surfaced in such magnitude in our society today. In my opinion there appears to be a correlation between more women entering the workforce and the increase of ADD children during the past 30 years.

I could be wrong, but let me explain why. I put my remarkable success down to my parents. My mother always knew everything about what I was doing and about me—listening in on phone calls, searching my room for drugs. She was always one step ahead of me. When I did fall over, my parents were always there to help me up and get me back on track. The same goes for schoolwork and homework. My parents were always probing my teachers and me to find out how I was going at school. They took the time to teach me to read and write. This is not uncommon but a lot of parents expect the school to do everything and it can't, especially with ADD children.

I am not suggesting that women should all quit their jobs and go back to being housewives. I am not saying that at all. The point I am trying to make is that children of today often do not have the same personal contact with their parents, as a result of longer working hours and our stressful lifestyle. The point I am making is that parents of ADD children must make a concerted effort to take the time with their children and have a more hands-on approach.

Why is ADD so wide spread in Australia and North America?

Many people whom I believe do not understand ADD allege that it is a disorder or condition invented by American drug companies. They believe that it is just another yuppie condition like chronic fatigue was presumed to be in the 1980s. These people think that ADD is now the yuppie condition of the 1990s. I refute this theory or assumption that it is a made-up condition. But the question still remains—why is ADD found in such large numbers in Australia and North America? There is a theory that attempts to answer this question and I believe it has some merits.

If we take a look at these two countries and especially their history, both are very similar. Australia and America were originally colonized in large numbers by immigrants who wanted a better life, and convicts. Hartmann asks the question, "What type of person would risk life and limb to travel thousands of miles to start a new life?" This type of person would have to be a risk taker, impulsive, forward thinking, and brash—the common characteristics of an ADD person.

Because ADD is hereditary, these two countries would have a larger percentage of ADD people in their short histories, so we can make the assumption that the large percentage of ADD cases in

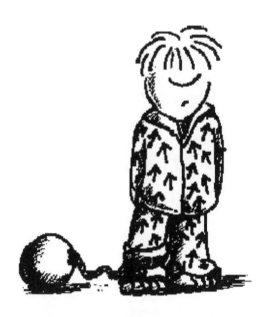

Australia and North America has a direct link with the men and women who colonized these great countries. With all these ADD genes being spread and passed along through the decades, it should not be a surprise to find that ADD is more common in these countries because it appears more often in our gene pool.

This assumption is made even stronger when you think about our culture compared to Britain's. Australians and Americans both have the view that the Brits are boring and very conservative. Conversely, Brits see Americans and Australians as loud, eccentric risk-takers. When you compare the English cricket team to the world champion Australian team, we can see a snapshot of both cultures and societies. The English team plays a defensive and risk-adverse style of cricket. On the other hand, the Australian team plays an exciting, attacking, high-risk style of cricket. This high-risk style of cricket can go two ways. It can end in a quick and decisive win, which is usually the case. Or they lose badly. The same goes for drawn matches. The recent Australian team hardly ever draws matches. They either win or lose. Conversely, England plays in many drawn matches and even plays for the draw.

To medicate or not to medicate? That is the question!

The issue of medication is one of the hottest topics in the ADD network. Parents are often extremely confused and concerned about the side effects of stimulant medication. Most parents and the media have no idea how it works or what it does. When I was younger I had some concerns about using Ritalin. When I was younger I blamed it for my height. The reason for this was I am only 165 cm (five foot six inches). I haven't grown since I was about fourteen. I laugh at this now because I am taller than both my parents, so I have come to the conclusion that it was not the medication but just genetics.

It makes me extremely angry when I hear in the media and from some doctors that medication is wrong and that we are breeding a generation of addicted children. The first thing parents must understand is that it is impossible to become addicted to this medication, even though, yes, it is dexamphetamine or, in an illegal drug, just plain old speed. This is where I feel the bad press about this medication comes from. But, unlike speed, it has a beneficial reaction on ADHD people.

How does dexamphetamine work?

Dexamphetamine is not a new drug. It has been used for many years. The only problem was that it was used for the wrong purpose. Dexamphetamine dates back to 1937. Dr Gordon

Serfontein in his book *The Hidden Handicap*, has said that in 1937, Dr. Bradley, a researcher in the United States, found some unusual results in his research with this new drug. He believed that it would relieve headaches in children subjected to pneumoencephalography. Pneumoencephalography is the technique of injecting air into a child's central nervous system. X-rays are taken to determine whether there is a tumor in the brain. This was later scrapped due to the development of CAT scans. The side effects of this were headaches after the procedure. Dr Bradley believed dexamphetamine might relieve these headaches.

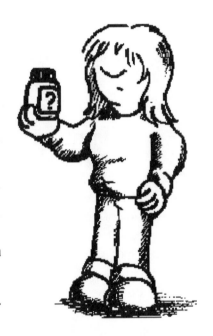

Bradley's studies did not show any improvement with headaches but did find that a number of children experiencing learning difficulties had substantial improvements in concentration and behavior and so on. As a result, dexamphetamine was further studied in the treatment of children with Minimal Brain Dysfunction, the first name given to children who suffered from Attention Deficit Disorder. A new drug was later released, methylphenidate (Ritalin), thought to be an improvement.

Serfontein said that there have been several long-term studies into the side-effects of this drug. The most interesting studies were in the 1950s by Dr. Weiss at the Montreal Children's Hospital over five years. There were three groups of children under investigation. The results showed some extremely interesting results in favor of dexamphetamine. A twenty-year follow-up study has not shown any long-term side effects.

To understand how dexamphetamine works, we need to get a little technical. ADD is the dysfunction of the neurotransmitter chemical that relays impulses from one cell to the next. The drug works by increasing the level of neurotransmitter in the gap between the two nerve cells.

Well, if you understood that, you are a whole lot smarter than I am because it took me a long time to grasp this concept. This is the reason I am writing this book—I am sick and tired of trying to understand all this medical mumbo jumbo in ADD books, especially when the books continually say, "We believe this" or "It is understood," etc. As best as I can work out, lots of doctors have lots of ideas on how they think ADD works. But no one knows for sure.

So how does it work, in English?

The brain works by sending electric impulses through brain cells. In a "normal" brain these impulses are sent and received undisturbed through brain cells. In an ADD brain these impulses are interrupted so the next cell does not receive the whole message. The medication basically increases these impulses so more messages are sent. It also limits the natural enzyme which destroys these messages.

Here's another way of looking at it: imagine the brain as a computer network sending email messages. With the ADD brain, when an email is sent only a quarter of the email is received by the next computer. The network cable is faulty because one of the wires is not connected properly. The medication basically sends more emails so that the whole email is understood. It also reconnects the faulty network wire, allowing the whole email to be sent to the next computer.

Side effects of stimulant medication

If anyone ever tells you that there are no side effects of stimulant medication, they are wrong. There are many, but how much they are felt and what types they are is different for every person. If you are wondering whether to use this medication you must first of all weigh up the pros and cons. If the side effects are very bad then of course you should not use the drug. But don't just dismiss it right away. There are a number of medications on the market and you should try all of them if necessary.

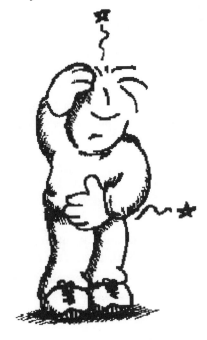

What are the side effects?

The known side effects of these drugs are only short term. There are no known long-term side effects. Short-term side effects are felt both during and after the medication has gone through your system. The longest lasting side effect is insomnia. This is a real issue with this medication, often missed because parents are not sleeping in the same room as their child. But I believe that the side effects do not outweigh the benefits of these drugs. I also believe that without these drugs I would not have succeeded as I have. Without these drugs I would not have passed secondary college and most likely would have ended up in a juvenile-detention center. And I wouldn't have been able to start writing this book, let alone finish it.

Here are other possible side effects:

> Appetite loss
> Fullness in the stomach
> Fatigue
> Headaches
> Dizziness
> Blurred vision
> Depression
> Irritability
> Increased tension
> Tearfulness

Only a couple of these side effects may be experienced by your child and usually only for a couple of months until your child's body adjusts to the medication.

The danger in medication is that parents feel that it is the answer to all their problems. Well, let me tell you, it is not. It only helps. Some people believe that medication will work straight away. This is not true. It takes months and months and even years. Remember my behavioral pattern in Year Seven? I was on medication and I was still the same old Ben. Within 12 months my behavior had changed drastically. I was a new kid, I had started to understand the way my brain worked. When I was on medication I started to understand how I was meant to behave. I also deliberately changed the way I thought. I tried at school and I tried to behave. It was not the medication, it was the better understanding of how my brain worked. But then in Year Nine I was still on medication and I chose to revert back to my old ways. No medication will change your

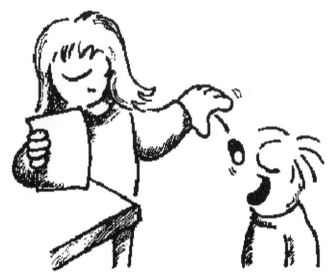

child overnight — it is a lifelong journey of learning to deal with ADD and how to control it.

When to medicate and not to medicate!

Some doctors believe that people like me should be medicated around the clock. I was at a conference in Sydney when a doctor made this ridiculous statement. It made me so angry. I feel this belief comes from our quick-fix society. Today when someone has a cold they go to the doctor and want a pill to fix it. Well, ADD can't be fixed with a pill. If someone out there does have a pill like this, please let me know! It would be most appreciated!

The first thing you must understand is that although medication is the best way to treat ADD, it does not solve it. I have heard of a mother medicating her son all day and then giving him a sleeping pill when he got home from school so she would not have to deal with him. I would like to meet this mother and ask her when is her son going to learn to deal with and understand his ADD if he is knocked out like a zombie all day and night? This is my argument against these powerful drugs. I am pro-medication—but only when you need it. Do you take headache tablets when you don't have a headache? No, of course you don't. So why do parents give their children these powerful drugs when they are behaving well? If you do this, your son never learns to deal with his ADD. Do you think when he turns eighteen and he moves out of home and stops taking his medication he is suddenly going to be able to control his erratic behavior?

I strongly believe that the only way to resolve ADD is to learn to deal with it. I know that is why I have done so well—not because I take Ritalin or because I saw a psychologist every week. It is because I learned to understand and develop practical strategies so I could function appropriately in society. I suggest that you medicate your child only when he needs it, usually at school and social functions. If your child is young, I can understand medicating him often. But as your child gets older he must learn to understand how to control his actions. People often think you grow out of ADD but this is not true—you just learn to control it.

The problems with over-medication!

This is the biggest problem with the issue of medication. The thing about taking so much medication both in dosages and over weeks without breaks is it makes your life a living hell. If you give your son too much medication it puts him into a zombie state. I hate this state and it makes me feel paranoid. I have often taken too much medication when doing homework and it's pretty scary. You go into a state of zombieness. I often find myself staring into

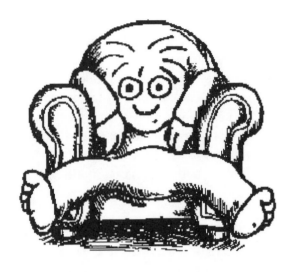

thin air concentrating on nothing. To do the simplest tasks seems impossible. I also find myself twitching and picking at my skin and I can't stop.

The problem with taking too much medication over a long period is that it drains your brain. You have to remember this medication makes you hyperfocus on things. So if you take it for weeks without breaks it is like extreme concentration for hours on end. Basically it's like over-working yourself when you're not doing anything. I have found when I take medication for long periods of time it creates the worst insomnia. I can be as drunk as a skunk and I just can't get to sleep. Along with this, it produces the worst headaches. I call these Ritalin headaches. These are often felt a couple of hours after the medication has worn off. This can be treated with a simple headache tablet.

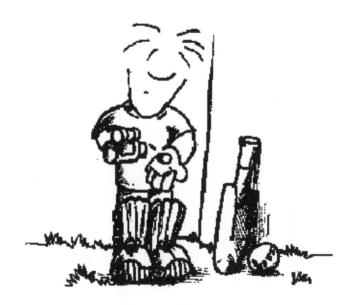

When to medicate?

The only time you should medicate your child is when he needs it. At school, it is often essential. I don't have a problem with this because I took it all the time at school. Other times are starting homework, family functions, while working, social events and playing sport. But it should never be taken on weekends unless really needed. Also, it should not be taken on school holidays. It's all about medication in moderation.

You must give your son time to recover after the school week. It is not a proven fact, but medication might cause reduced growth due to reduced appetite. However, there may also be other causes that we don't know yet. This is believed to be due to lack of food at an age when your son is doing his growing. So it is very important to give your son plenty of breaks from medication to allow his height to catch up.

As well, when you take too much medication over a long period of time its effects are not as great. It will save you money not to medicate too much because you will not have to increase the dosage.

Taking too much medication over a long period of time also produces counter-productive results. If your son takes too much medication it drains his body physically and especially mentally. When he is coming down off the medication he is mentally exhausted. The slightest thing may trigger a violent or erratic outburst.

You should never give your son medication when he is doing nothing. It may make your life easier but it is just cruel. When your son is on medication his brain is over-stimulated and is in hyper mode. He is thinking frantically and must be stimulated either by physical or mental means. If your son is on medication you must give him things to do. If he is just sitting in front of the television he is just hyper-focusing on a box. Ever wondered why your son is twitching and so fidgety when he is on medication? It is because he is mentally unstimulated. By rubbing and picking his skin he is hyper-focusing on that. Not a very nice experience, I can tell you.

How should medication be taken?

Medication should be taken by your child. It is all right for you to hand it to them but they must learn to take it themselves. It should be taken with food because this releases it more slowly. If I take it without food it hits me like a hammer and I go straight into a zombie state. In my experience, it takes about forty minutes to feel any effects. Around an hour and a half after medication has been taken the greatest effects are being felt. You should tell your child why he is taking it and how it improves his behavior,

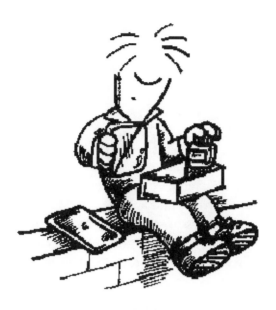

concentration and so on. I suggest filming him when he is on medication and when he is not. This will help him understand the appropriate way to act. And when he is not acting appropriately he will learn to self-medicate, which is extremely important as he gets older.

The biggest problem with your son self-medicating himself is at school. My dosage was two tablets in the morning and two tablets at lunch. My mother would put my tablets in my lunch box and I was meant to take them. But the medication reduced my appetite. I would not eat my lunch and not take my tablets. This was a real problem for me because I would always play up at the end of the day. A lot of schools demand that ADD students go to the office to take their medication. This is all right when your son is young but it also makes him feel different and again reinforces his low self-esteem.

As your son gets older I suggest that he should be responsible for his own medication. If he does not take it, he is the only one he is going to hurt. I also don't like the idea of an eighteen-year-old student going off to take his medication like a little school kid. Come on, we are talking about adults.

How to choose the right school for your child!

The right or wrong school can be the determining factor in the level of success your child achieves in both school and in life. Without the right choices of schools my parents made, I would not have succeeded. You must make the right choice of school for your child because it will help him resolve many of the problems caused by ADD.

To choose the right school you must first know what makes a good school for an ADD student. The first thing you need to look at is its size. I suggest the smallest school possible, with small classes. This will allow your child to have more one-on-one teaching. This is essential if your child is having trouble academically. The smaller classes also have a more settled working environment. This will help your child's concentration. In small schools the teachers often have more time to give to each student and there is a more caring environment.

Once you have found a small school, I suggest asking about any special education programs. Just come straight out and say it. "Does your school and do your teachers have any experience in dealing with ADHD students?" If they do, ask them what? Find out about their sporting and drama programs. This will be of great help for your child to burn off their excess energy.

A good question is, "Does your school offer any big brother (older student) programs?" These are great for ADD students. It

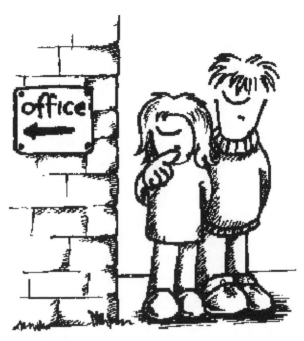

offers them a service of remedial schooling with one-on-one teaching. It is amazing how much an ADD student will listen to an older student. The next thing you want to find out is how many male teachers the school has. This may sound extremely sexist but in my experience male ADD students relate best to male teachers because they can handle a lot more boisterous behavior.

For ADD children I believe the best types of schools are same-sex religious schools only because they have a higher standard of discipline and your child will need plenty of discipline to keep his behavior under control. Public schools are disadvantaged when some parents will not allow teachers to discipline their unruly children. I am not religious but my parents felt that these schools would be the best and they were right for me.

After all this has been done, you must make a list of all the schools that you feel would be beneficial for your child. I strongly suggest that you take your son to all these schools on the list and let him decide. Then it is his decision and he can't turn around and blame you if he does not like the school.

For your son, try to get a male teacher. This may be hard with the shortage of male teachers in Australia, but do try.

A lot of ADD students are kept down in the younger years. I think this is the worst thing you can do. Sure, your child may be academically behind. But in early years, who really cares? It will take years before your child catches up. The reason I don't like ADD students staying down is that it does so much harm to their self-confidence and causes further problems. You have to remember that your child is most probably extremely gifted in some area, like many ADD people. But it takes many years for an ADD student to learn how to study in their own manner. We can concentrate, we just do it when we feel like it. So when your child realizes this, the results will astound both of you. Some of the greatest minds in history have shown many traits of ADD. These people often had trouble in school, but when alone they could develop some remarkable results. According to Dr. Gordon Serfontein in his book *ADD in Adults*, Albert Einstein had every ADD symptom under the sun.

What to do if the school has had enough of your child!

Well, this is definitely my forte because I went to six schools. About every two years I had to find another school. Some parents often have real trouble with changing schools a lot. But it is not a real problem. It can be really beneficial. As they say, a change is as good as a holiday. If your child really hates the school,

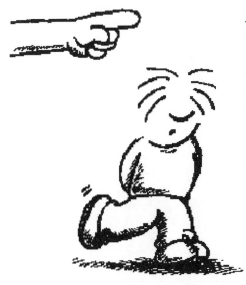

just pull them out and try again. But what do you do when the school has had enough? In most cases you can't do a lot. But if you want him to stay at the school, just ask them, "What is going to happen to my son if you expel him? Are you just going to move the problem on? I thought schools are meant to care about the youth of this country. Well, I guess I was wrong."

The only thing that really matters is that your son is happy at school. If he is upset just pull him out. Try, try, try again. If he is just not going to make it at school, home schooling is always an option. Tutors are also great because your son can catch up working at home in a more stable environment. The one thing parents must realize is that not all kids will end up to be rocket scientists. If your son is not going to make it academically, when appropriate, ask him if he would like to try a trade school or maybe an apprenticeship. He may be better at manual skills than academic theory. It's worth a try. As long as he is happy, who really cares? Not everyone can go or wants to go to university.

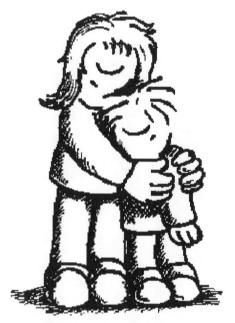

Relationships

Mother-son relationship

This is the most important relationship an ADD child can have. I know I would not have achieved anything in life without my mother. Thanks, Mum! The reason this relationship is so important is the mother does everything for an ADD kid. Mothers often say, "I do everything, he is so lazy." It's why this relationship is so important. Mothers are the stabilizers of a family and they have a calming effect on an ADD child. Mothers must understand that it does not matter how much your child abuses you, he still loves you. I have already explained why mothers often get the abuse and violence directed at them. My mother still does everything for me, which sounds pretty sad. But without this my life would just be a scattered mess.

Father-son relationship

This is a very important relationship. When kids are young they idolize their fathers and they want to be just like them. This all changes when they get older. Fathers must play a key role in raising an ADD child. They have all those little father-son chats about life and so on. Fathers also give great guidance and can point you in the right direction. But when the father does not put any effort into raising the child it makes it really hard for the mother. Dads are good for doing all the energetic stuff with your son as well.

The problem arises time and time again when the father gets home from a long day at work and the last thing he wants to hear is, "Our son did this and did that." The son is often excited about their dad being home and wants to play. The father often shuts all this out and leaves it to his wife to deal with. The father then stays at work more and more so he does not have to deal with it. This puts massive strain on the marriage and many ADD children's parents break up due to this constant pressure. I cannot stress how important it is for fathers to make an effort with their sons because it really makes a difference in the overall success of your son.

Sibling relationships

This is a very hard relationship for both the siblings and the ADD child. ADD children are prone to annoy and frustrate their brothers and sisters. It is even further aggravated when they go to the same school. The siblings are often made to stand out for bad things their brother (or sister) has done. As well, this is a very hard relationship to achieve good results in because the ADD child often gets most of the attention from the parents. This makes it extremely hard on the other siblings because they resent and are often jealous of the special treatment the ADD child gets.

I suggest that you explain to your other children what is wrong with their brother and even go as far as telling their friends. This is all about understanding and awareness and when people understand that ADD children can't help the way they behave a lot of the stigma about being a bad kid is wiped away.

Lots of family meetings are a good way to resolve issues that would often otherwise end up in fights. You can't make your children like each other but you can reduce the tension.

Another great idea is to ask a older cousin, one who your child looks up to, to spend time with your son. Children mimic the behavior of older kids and this can be a good way to show your child the right way to behave. Even getting an older cousin to tutor your child can be very beneficial.

Student-teacher relationship

This relationship can be so beneficial for your child. It is of the utmost importance to explain to your son's teacher why he acts the way he does. This will give your son more of a chance to bend the rules without getting into trouble. The most important thing about a good student-teacher relationship is mutual respect. If your son hates the teacher he will do everything in his power to annoy the teacher. But if your son likes his teacher the teacher will be able to control your son better because he sees the teacher as a friend. In Year Twelve my coordinator always wondered why I never got into trouble in Economics but was in trouble in every other class. I told her that it was simple. I liked the teacher and if he asked me to be quiet or do my work I would, because I didn't want to disappoint him. But I didn't like the other teachers as much, so I went out of my way to highlight this through disruptive behavior.

Parent-teacher relationships must be established. A good

relationship will help your child. A couple of chats a week will help in the understanding of both the teacher's responsibility and your child's. It is great to find out what work is due. ADD students often forget about homework and dates. Once you have found out what is due and when, you should make a huge sign in your child's room to give them a constant reminder of when work is due. Once it is done, get your child to cross it off and give them a reward for completing the set tasks on time.

Lazy child!

I am constantly being told by my parents, "You don't do anything. You're so lazy, Ben!" This is a common trait in ADD people. It contradicts the name "Attention Deficit Hyperactivity Disorder." If I am meant to be hyperactive, how can I be lazy? It is not that we are deliberately lazy, we just have short bursts of energetic behavior. This is then followed by many hours, even days, of complete nothingness. It is not uncommon for me to study for twelve hours straight then do nothing for days and lie in bed. It seems as if there can't be a mixture of the two.

Being lazy is a condition of ADD. People with ADD do not choose to be lazy but cannot concentrate on one thing at a time. They are constantly trying to will themselves on to do things. But they just can't motivate themselves to do it.

How to teach an ADD child!

This is a huge problem for parents of children who have ADD. How can you teach a child who can't concentrate and is not interested in the subject being taught? I believe that the problem with many ADD children is not that they do not want to learn, because many ADD children are hungry to gain knowledge. But the way they are taught is not appropriate for their brain pattern. Many parents spend thousands of dollars on learning aids to help their children, but they don't work because these learning tools have been developed for normal children. This problem again arises in the classroom. The teacher tries to teach the class with learning styles taught in teacher's college. But they have no idea how to teach an ADD child. It does not matter how much you try to teach an ADD child in the normal teaching style, they will gain nothing. This took me many years to understand but when I did I could teach myself.

So how do ADD students learn?

The first thing we must look at is why the old style of teaching is not appropriate for ADD children. The problem with the old style is that it does not capture the imagination and the low concentration of ADD students. How can you expect to teach a child math when it means nothing to them? What I am saying here is that when you open a math textbook it is full of sums and numbers. It means nothing to an ADD child. Conversely, a normal child is told that he must do these sums and hand in his homework the following day. He can do this because he does not have a problem with concentration and repetitive tasks.

This is the same problem with reading. I recently did a talk for a group of Year Eight ADD students who were failing at school. I asked them, "Who likes to read books?" Not one person said they did. I asked why. They said, "Because it is boring," and some said they couldn't read anyway. I related to this predicament so well. I have a thirst for knowledge but the only way you can get a good knowledge of a topic is to read many accounts of the topic. This was always a problem for me. Only recently I learnt why I can't read for long periods. This will be extremely useful for many ADD students.

How to teach an ADD student to read!

It was only a few months ago I read my first book cover to cover. While reading this book it occurred to me why I could not concentrate when reading books. It was not that I did not find the material interesting. It was that I was just reading words. If you pick up a book written in another language it is just a bunch of paper with symbols on it. That is the problem with books for ADD people. When I was younger I would complain that I would read a couple of pages and them forget what I had read. How could I understand a story if I could only remember 5 percent of it? Talking to other ADD people, they too felt the same way.

The only way an ADD student can read for long periods of time is to forget that they are reading words. The best way to do this is to become part of the book. I suggest choosing a character and becoming that character throughout the novel. Instead of reading a book, you are now experiencing and living the book. Instead of reading the book and the book telling you what you are thinking you must think outside the book. It is like having your own movie screen in your mind. When your character chooses to do something in the novel you must visualize the scene in your mind. Then ask yourself what you would do in the same situation.

There are a number of books on the market for teenage readers where you choose your own destiny. You decide which way you will go with the book or story. How it works is at the end of each chapter you have the chance to choose from three scenarios. You then flip to that page and continue reading. These books are excellent because you must become a part of the book without actually doing it. The only problem with these books is that at times they can become a little confusing to understand when you are constantly flipping the pages. Overall, these books can be very useful.

How to teach young ADD students to learn how to read!

This is a major problem for both parents and students who have ADD. The problem with teaching young ADD students is that they have short-term memory problems. I often become annoyed with trying to teach young ADD students to read. One minute they can read a word then the next minute they have forgotten it.

To teach an ADD child to learn the first 100 words or so of the English language is the most important thing. However, these words are often the hardest to remember and read. For example, it is extremely hard to try to tell an ADD child to read the word "what" because when you sound the word it sounds "wot." Most children can learn the first 100 words of the English language by continually repeating and doing lines of the words but this is not possible with an ADD student. Once an ADD child has read the word he does not want to continually read and spell the word so it is firmly stuck in his mind. Therefore learning modifications and techniques must be adapted.

The best way to teach an ADD student to learn words is not by normal teaching techniques. You must develop your own techniques for each situation. For example: if your child is interested in basketball you can play a game of HORSE. This is an excellent game for fathers to play with their son. How it works is each time you make a shot you get a letter. So if you make your first shot you receive the letter H and as you follow the key around and make shots you get more letters until you have spelled the word HORSE. You can then do this with other words such as "what," "where," "who," "the," "that," and so on. If learning is made fun your child will want to learn. If you try to force your child to learn you will only achieve a little success.

The learning technique can be also be used when teaching math. You pick a sport such as football, cricket, basketball and so on depending on your child's interests. Cricket is a good game to choose. Make sure your son bats second or it will not work as well. The first team bats and makes a score of 150 runs. Then your son has to bat. But beforehand your son must do some small calculations. For example:

Your son needs 151 runs to win off 25 overs with ten batsmen remaining. So how many runs per over is needed to win and what average does each batsman need to make for the team to win?

151 runs divided by 25 overs = run rate required

or

151/25 = 6.04

Run rate required is : 6.04

What is the average of each batsman needed to win?

151/10 =15.1

Average needed is : 15.1 runs

These simple mathematical problems are extremely useful for your son when he is faced with the same problems in the classroom. As well as this, you should make your son count his own running score of runs. This will help with his short-term memory and learning retention. These sums should also be done during and after the game. This will teach him to think ahead and plan for the future, something that is very hard for ADD kids to do.

Once your young ADD child has learned the first 100 words of the English language it is now time for them to start to put these into sentences. The same learning techniques as HORSE can be used in the same way. They will just have to make sentences instead of spelling words. Once they can make sentences it is time for them to read books. This will again be tough to do. But with modification it should be much easier. The best way to do this is to find books that your son is interested in, for example on sports, music, cars and so on. If he has trouble keeping an interest in books you could use another source. When I was learning to read I hated reading books. However I was very interested in Teenage Mutant

Ninja Turtles, a craze then. My parents would buy me Turtle trading cards. On the backs of these cards there was a short story. I read the backs of the cards instead of books. These cards are extremely useful because they have short stories and pictures on both the front and backs of the card. They capture the short attention span of ADD children.

Another modification that I suggest is visual reading. You find a book that your son is interested in and change it slightly. This may be very time-consuming but it is very effective. You will need to go out and buy a CD-ROM that has clip art pictures on it. You can also download these pictures from the Net. You will then need to re-type the story on your PC. But every five to ten words instead of writing the word place the picture of the word. Then type the word under the picture. For example, place the word 'fire engine' under a picture of a fire engine. This learning technique works in the same way as adapting a character in a novel. It is all about visual learning and stimulation.

Another modification is color coding word groups, for example "cat," "bat," "that," "mat," and so on. But color code only the "at" sound. If you do this in a number of books your son will visually learn the words. Writing the first 100 words on flash cards in color coding is a good tool. The problem is people use these flash cards in the wrong way. Many parents stick these cards on walls, doors and so on. They then ask their son to read the cards but this is impossible. How can they expect their son to read the words when there are another 99 cards distracting their concentration? The flash cards should be used in another way. You should hold the cards right up in the face of your son. This way the only thing he will be able to concentrate on is that specific word. Then get your son to read that card. Because the cards are color-coded he will again reinforce the color of the word with the sound. This will work at the start but once your son can read most of the words he will become bored. The best way to resolve this problem is to use sporting heroes and dirty words and stories. By placing pictures of sporting heroes, cars and so on it again creates visual interest with your son. Once your son can read most of the words it is time to use dirty words to create interest, for example, "grass," "glass," "fast," "ass!" You will be surprised at how much interest a seven year old will have when he reads the word "ass."

Telling stories with these flash cards is a fantastic way of retaining interest. All you need to do is ask your son to read the word and then put that word into a story. He then chooses the next word and puts it into the story. It is a good idea to make the story involve your son and a sporting hero and dirty words. He will be constantly laughing and will want more and more. He won't even notice that he is learning.

Short term memory modifications

The game of memory is an excellent way to improve short-term memory. It works by placing playing cards down and trying to find the matching pair. It is a very simple game but works very well. This should be used frequently in younger children because it is of the utmost importance to improve this at a young age.

Many people and teachers have been astounded by my incredible long-term memory. But at the same time they cannot understand my poor short-term memory. This is a huge problem for me when trying to cram for exams. For many months I thought about why I have such a good long-term memory, and then it hit me. I don't remember things but I remember features of stories that I find amusing or interesting. For example, if I had to remember the 6th of August 1945 when Japan surrendered to the Allies at the end of World War II, I would not have a chance in hell. But what I do subconsciously is picture in my mind the massive mushroom cloud over Hiroshima when the atomic bomb was detonated. What I

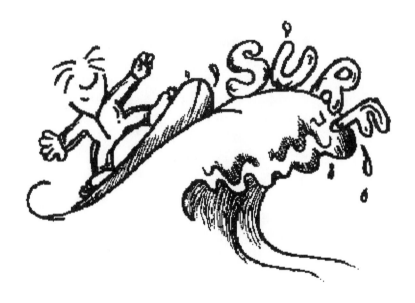

visualize is the date "6th of August 1945" being exploded instead.
So when I need to remember the date all I need to do is visualize
the mushroom cloud and the date pops into my head.

Another example is trying to teach an ADD child to spell the
word "surf." This is very hard to explain to an ADD child and is
most useful when they are around twelve. To remember the word
surf you must visualize yourself surfing on the perfect wave. But
just then a huge S on a surfboard cuts you off. U, R, F are surfing
past as well so follow this. When your son needs to remember how
to spell the word "surf" all he needs to do is jump on his imaginary
surfboard in his mind and the word will suddenly pop into his
mind.

I understand that this is very hard to explain to a child and even
some adults. But once you have mastered this memory technique
you will be astounded with your new memory. It works by visually
triggering a subtle cue in your mind. I think of my memory as being
a bit like my room. I know that my keys are in it somewhere but I

can't remember where. We have all looked for something and been unable to find it. But suddenly you remember something and it triggers your memory where you put it. That is how this technique works. It allows you to remember strange and funny things and to remember boring and dull things like dates and numbers.

Homework!

Homework is one of the hardest things to try and get an ADD student to do. I have always hated doing homework and I never did any substantial homework until I got to Year Twelve. It was during this period that I learned a lot more about myself and how my brain works. I have already discussed how I do my homework but that is me. I will now discuss how you can try to make your child do homework on a regular basis.

The first thing you must do is make homework fun. Do not make it a chore or a punishment. You must encourage your son to want to learn. This can only be done by motivation. Firstly, all subjects must be organized into color-coded folders, English being red, history being blue and so on. Each folder should have a picture of a favorite sporting star or hero on the front. When your son gets older, pictures of models and sexy movie stars can be used. Homework must be done at the same time every night and start and finish at the same time. When it is time to do homework instead of saying, "Get your red English homework folder," you should say "Get your Michael Jordan folder." This takes away the negativity of doing homework from the start. Along with this, you can use bribery and treats to motivate, for example sticking treats on the folder. This again makes doing homework enjoyable.

Trying to make an ADD student do something when he is not

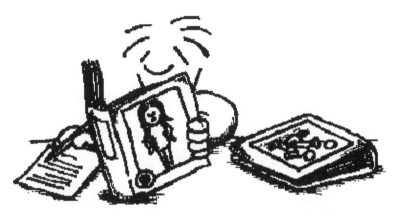

mentally ready to do it makes it very hard for parents. Most people don't understand that sometimes an ADD person can be perfectly capable of doing homework and the next day can't concentrate on the simplest tasks. This is a common problem for me. One day I can concentrate and then the next I can't concentrate on anything. Some days I am lazy and can't move. But then the next I am so hyper I can't sit still. When something needs to be done like homework I can't mentally do it. I can't concentrate.

I have overcome this problem with exercise and energetic behavior. If I feel that I am too hyper and can't sit still I go and do something energetic before I sit still and do homework. This feeling of hyperactivity often comes back when doing homework and when I feel this coming on I know that it is time to do something energetic. I often just get up and walk out of my room and go and swing a golf club. It takes only a couple of minutes and I am fine and ready to study again. This was a problem in class because I could not just walk out and swing a golf club. Parents and teachers need to be aware of this and let the ADD student just walk off and come back in a couple of minutes. Teachers can do it subtly by getting the ADD student to go and run a note to another teacher on the other side of the school. All the note needs to say is that so and so needs a break.

In Year Twelve my mother had bought a straw hat from an opportunity shop for a dress-up party. This hat became my homework hat in Year Twelve. Every time I started homework I would put the hat on. This visual cue told my brain that it was time to do homework. Once I stopped it came off or when I went outside to swing the golf club. I still have the hat today but it is destroyed because I would throw it across the room when I was sick of doing homework. I plan to keep it forever.

Another excellent aid for ADD students is the personal computer. If I did not have a computer, I would not have achieved anything. ADD children often have many problems with spelling and writing. The computer helps ADD people who have trouble in these areas. The spell check is the greatest thing invented. A word-processing program is even better. It allows an ADD person to express their ideas and thoughts so other people can read them. If I had written this book with a pen, I couldn't have even read my own writing and I guess my editor would have had no chance.

The PC is most useful for ADD people when it is away from the family. It allows an ADD child to work quietly without distractions. For parents, it is also useful as an escape and a learning aid. The Internet often attracts ADD people because it allows them to absorb lots of different information. When they are bored or not interested in that topic any more all they need to do is find something else. The PC can also help with schoolwork. There are heaps of good learning games on the market that provide visual stimulation and the challenge increases with ability. They are also predominately used by one person. The PC becomes an ADD person's own personal tutor.

The other thing about homework is that parents and students should discuss with their teacher if it is possible to choose the topic of the assignment. This can be very useful for ADD students because if they pick a topic they are interested in they will have

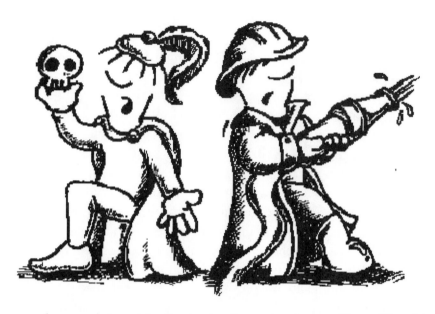

much more interest in the topic. Some teachers will not like this idea. But it is narrow-minded teachers like this who cause a lot of problems for ADD students. In my opinion it does not matter what your son learns as long as he is learning something. Once he is older and understands how his own mind works it will not matter. But in younger ADD students it is very important for them to learn something about anything. Knowledge is power and the key to many doors.

ADD jobs and careers

People with ADD often find themselves either hating their job or swapping between jobs all the time. Statistics show that ADD people change jobs three times more often than the average. This is a result of being easily bored and unstimulated in the workplace. On a personal note, I am constantly swapping part-time jobs because I either get bored and play up and get fired or I just leave. My biggest problem is that I have a major problem with authority. This is not a good trait when you are sixteen and tell your boss that he is stupid. But that's me!

Around two years ago I decided, or realized, that I was not going to be able to work for anyone but myself, as a result of my authority issue and thinking most bosses are just stupid. They're not, but I just can't handle being told what to do. Therefore I decided that I should stop doing a Bachelor of Business in Administration and start a Bachelor of Business in Entrepreneurial Studies. My theory is that if I am going to be fired, it is better to fire myself.

However, this is not appropriate in all cases. So I have suggested some jobs that I think are appropriate for ADD people. Obviously there are many other suitable jobs. The most unsuitable is any job that is repetitive and/or boring. The ADD person will not stay in a boring job. The key issue in all these careers is constant stimulation and excitement. But, more importantly, they allow ADD people to work by themselves without being restricted by their employers.

Author
Professional athlete
Computer technology
Real estate agent
Stock broker
Plumber
Builder
Electrician
Actor
Entrepreneur
The army
Police force
Fire fighter
Advertising
Politician

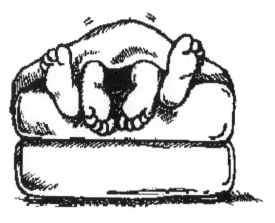

Sex

ADD people are at more risk of contracting sexually transmitted diseases compared to the normal population. This is a result of taking risks when having sex by not using protection. ADD people are sometimes described as sex maniacs. But this is a huge generalization. I believe that the reason some ADD people like to have sex a lot is not because they are slutty. The reason, I feel, is that ADD people live off the excitement of sex.

However, the problem still remains that ADD people are more likely to contract sexually transmitted diseases than the norm. Also, teenage pregnancy is an issue for ADD girls. Parents must realize that your children are going to have sex and you can't stop it. But you must do all you can to protect your child. Sex education at school is not enough any more. Parents must take an active role and explain the risks, and the other alternatives to unprotected sex.

Interesting statistics about ADHD adolescents

From ADHD in the Third Millennium Conference held at Westmead Hospital, Sydney, Australia. March 16–18, 2001, p.98

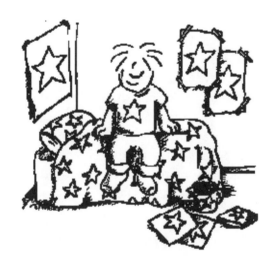

Begin sexual activity 1 year earlier (14–15 yrs).
More sexual partners/less time with each.
Less likely to employ contraception.
38% have teen pregnancies (vs. 4%).
54% do not have custody of offspring.
16% treated for STDs (vs. 4%).
Greater use of alcohol and marijuana.
Greater risk for cardiovascular disease.

Obsessions and fads

Obsessions and fads are more commonly experienced by younger ADD people. Fads can often drive parents crazy—having to be constantly told about something until they too are experts in that field. I personally put my parents through the Teenage Mutant Ninja Turtles University until I got over it around four years later. Obsessions are even more annoying for parents—for example, becoming fixated with disliking a teacher or a relative. I don't think that it is often the actual person or television program that causes the obsession, but the excitement and feeling of aliveness that young ADD people get when their obsession or fad is discussed or seen.

Parents should not try to prevent these fads and obsessions. They can be a very useful tool in the classroom. Instead of viewing it as a disadvantage, use it as an advantage. See if you can involve your child's fad into every day life as much as possible when it comes to getting him to do boring tasks such as homework, cleaning his room, etc. He will show more interest if his fad or obsession is linked directly to the unstimulating tasks.

Lessons from history

I once hated history and thought it was a waste of time. I didn't care what had happened before me. I am a now person—what was happening now was all that mattered. Then one day I asked my history teacher. "What do we need history for?" The reply was: "To predict the future, we must first understand the past!" It sounded good but I didn't quite understand it until I was much older. There is one certain thing on this planet and that is there has been nothing new. It has all happened before with a few changes. Countries, armies, leaders, diseases, miracles, all come and go. The same goes for people and especially ADD people. What parents are dealing with now with their ADD children has been happening for thousands of years. There are many well-known famous people suspected of having ADD. I would love to write about them but I can't because I face the possibility of being sued. If you are interested, all you need to do is search for 'famous ADD people' on the Internet. You will be surprised at first then when you think about them it will make a lot of sense. Therefore, I will discuss two famous ADD people. The interesting thing I have found in researching famous ADD people is that many of these people failed at school, but they succeeded in life. As already discussed, it's not easy for ADD people of today to succeed without a good education. The other interesting thing I have found is that these famous ADD people were all brilliant. But at the same time they would seem very mad and crazy to non-ADD people. As the saying goes, "It's a very fine line between brilliance and utter madness." This basically describes me to a T. My mother often says, "How can someone so intelligent be so stupid?"

The king of ADD! Winston Churchill

Dr Serfontein's book *ADD in Adults* has said that as a young boy, Winston Churchill showed all the characteristics of ADD. He was a very mischievous boy who was always in trouble and antagonizing people. Winston's mother often complained to his father that he was always teasing his younger brother. Winston said himself that he was "what grown up people in their off-hand way call a troublesome boy."

He had major problems at school, especially in his early school days. He was described as a daydreamer and could never stay on task. His school work and homework were never completed on time and hardly even done. His poor attention in the classroom got him into a lot of trouble. He was disorganized and constantly late for class. His adventurous nature could be seen in his early days. His parents did not know what would happen to him and if he would amount to anything.

However, like many ADD people who show early signs of achieving little, he showed the world what can be achieved when you put your mind to it. When he finished school he joined the army and traveled the world. He fought in many wars and conflicts across the globe. He had many near-death experiences as a result of his impulsiveness and sometimes stupid behavior. He has been described as very brave. I do not feel that he was so brave but more impulsive and didn't think about the consequences—a common trait in ADD people. Many brave acts have been later described as complete craziness and stupidity. These brave people realize afterwards how dangerous it was. However, the fact still remains that he did perform some very brave deeds and he should be respected and honored for them.

In his army days he recognized his fascination and ability as a writer and more importantly as a speechmaker. When he left the army, he followed his abilities in these fields and became one of the greatest politicians the world has ever seen. Like many ADD people, he had an ability to grasp very complex problems quickly. This was one of his major strengths when leading the Allies to victory against the Nazis. When Churchill was handed long reports on the war he was not able to concentrate to read all the pages. Therefore he was given simplified one to two page reports—what we know today as an executive summary. What was more important than Churchill's ability to grasp impossible concepts in a matter of minutes was his ability to translate and communicate them to the general public.

His impulsive nature and ability to understand complex problems was a key factor in defeating the Germans. He was able to understand the problem and then act upon it as soon as possible. This impulsiveness sometimes ended in horrific disaster, especially during the war. But most of the time it was dramatically successful.

The one thing that made Churchill such a success was not his family or even his ADD—it was that he learned to control his erratic behavior. This was developed by his upbringing. In his early days and early twenties, he was in a restricted environment—school and the army. ADD people need routine, and the institutions Winston attended were based on routine. Later in life, he adopted these skills himself. Without this early training, I do not feel he would have been such a success.

Albert Einstein

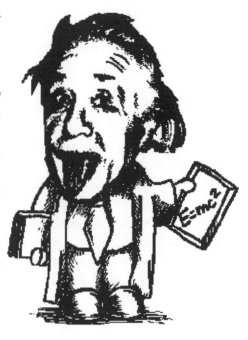

Dr Serfontein also discussed Albert Einstein in his book *ADD in Adults*. Einstein was best known for his theory of relativity. But he was also respected as the founder of contemporary science and physics theory. His theories are still fundamentally important to today's scientific approaches. The later development of the atomic bomb can also be attributed to his research, although he disagreed with its development and use. When Einstein was twelve he came to the assumption that a personal god did not exist. This allowed him to free himself from the spiritual and ethical restrictions of being a believer. As a young boy, Einstein had learning difficulties. At age four he could speak only two-word sentences. As a result of his late development he was believed perhaps to be mentally retarded. His tremendous difficulties at school were attributed to his poor concentration. In class he was always thinking about things other than what was being taught. The two things he could concentrate on, though, were arithmetic and science.

Einstein dropped out of school but continued to study on his own. When his father's business failed he had to find employment and support himself. Einstein thought that he would excel at electrical engineering and attempted to study at the Swiss Federal Polytechnics School, but he failed the general entrance exam. However, he scored very highly on the mathematics section and they suggested that he work for a diploma at the Swiss High School and reapply. He did and was accepted the following year.

Like Winston Churchill, Albert Einstein's true ability was to break down complex problems into smaller parts. This is how he solved some of modern man's most complex mathematical and scientific equations.

Einstein was not an angry and violent ADD person. That can be the case with some ADD people. He was more of the inattentive and easily distracted type. Einstein's success, like Winston Churchill's, was due to him being able to control his concentration through a deliberate and ordered life. Similar to his ability to disregard the clutter of mathematical problems and reach the core of the problem, Einstein was able to free his mind of clutter and concentrate on his research and studies.

Conclusion

Writing this book is my greatest achievement to date. It took many long months to write and I just hope that all my hard work will help other people to understand ADD—and more importantly, their children—better. The most important thing all parents must keep in mind is that hard work is the only way for your child to survive in this world. A parent's love and understanding is the greatest gift you can give to your child. Along with this, patience and an open mind will help your family function in a more normal manner.

If I had not had my strong family support I would have not achieved anything. I would have ended up just another statistic, a juvenile ADD person in jail. However, I did have strong family support and look at what I achieved as a result.

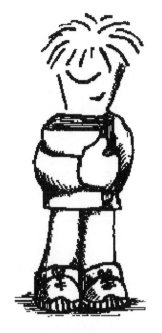

Hope is the best gift I can give parents and children with ADD. I have severe ADHD, which resulted in me going to six different schools, but my parents and I never gave up and I finally made it through the school system. Now I am studying at one of the best universities in Australia. Who would have thought that a person with a diagnosed mental and learning disability would make it to university? Most people don't know that I can't spell properly, let alone read my own handwriting. But like other skills I lack, I have learned to work around them. It sounds stupid that a person who can't spell can write a book, because I have. But what sounds even more ridiculous is someone writing a book who has only ever read one book before. It sounds and it is ridiculous, but I did. I am not trying to boast. I am just stating that anything is possible if you put your mind to it!

In the future I plan to write another book that will focus on how to teach ADD children and how to survive through university/college. I hope this book will help educate teachers and parents to learn how to teach ADD students. I feel that the current school system is restricting some of our brightest young people by not reaching them in the classroom. Many ADD students are wasted talents because they do not reach their full potential as a result of not achieving in the classroom and school system.

On a closing note, I would like to thank everyone who purchased and read my book. If you got this far, you obviously thought it was worth reading. I hope that you found it informative and you now understand ADD and your child better than before you read it. I wish you and your child the greatest success in this sometimes crazy world.

Always remember to reach for the stars!

Best wishes,
Benjamin Polis